U0297500

中药炮制学实验与指导

Experiment and Guide for Processing of Chinese Herb Medicine

第3版

（供中药学、中药资源与开发、中药制药学、药学及相关专业用）

主　　编　张春凤

英文主编　潘荣杰

主　　审　杨中林

副主编　李　飞　季　德　杨小林

编　　委　（以姓氏笔画为序）

马志国（暨南大学药学院）　　　孙小雅（中国药科大学）

李　飞（中国药科大学）　　　　李　凯（河南中医药大学）

李兴华（中国药科大学）　　　　杨小林（上海中医药大学）

张春凤（中国药科大学）　　　　陆奕霜（中国药科大学）

陈玉江（中国药科大学）　　　　季　德（南京中医药大学）

赵雅兰（中国药科大学）　　　　徐　健（中国药科大学）

郭常润（中国药科大学）　　　　曹衡健（中国药科大学）

颜家壬（中国药科大学）　　　　薛鹏飞（中国药科大学）

秘　　书　孙小雅（中国药科大学）

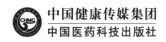

中国健康传媒集团

中国医药科技出版社

内 容 提 要

本教材是"全国高等医药院校药学类专业第三轮实验双语教材"之一。本教材共包括净制、切制、炒法、炙法、煅法、蒸法、煮法、燀法和其他方法等23个实验，既有传统实验技能的训练，又采用现代技术方法对传统炮制理论的验证，理论联系实际，实用性强。本教材适用于全日制中药学、中药资源与开发、中药制药学、药学等相关专业师生教学使用，亦可作为医药院校、职业院校药学专业或医药人员及中药炮制实验技术人员参考资料。

图书在版编目（CIP）数据

中药炮制学实验与指导：汉英对照/张春凤主编.— 3 版.—北京：中国医药科技出版社，2023.11

全国高等医药院校药学类专业第三轮实验双语教材

ISBN 978-7-5214-4277-9

Ⅰ.①中… Ⅱ.①张… Ⅲ.①中药炮制学 – 实验 – 双语教学 – 医学院校 – 教学参考资料 – 汉、英 Ⅳ.① R283-33

中国国家版本馆 CIP 数据核字（2023）第 202355 号

美术编辑 陈君杞

版式设计 友全图文

出版 **中国健康传媒集团** | 中国医药科技出版社

地址 北京市海淀区文慧园北路甲 22 号

邮编 100082

电话 发行：010-62227427 邮购：010-62236938

网址 www.cmstp.com

规格 889 × 1194 mm $^1/_{16}$

印张 8 $^1/_2$

字数 230 千字

初版 2003 年 8 月第 1 版

版次 2023 年 11 月第 3 版

印次 2023 年 11 月第 1 次印刷

印刷 北京盛通印刷股份有限公司

经销 全国各地新华书店

书号 ISBN 978-7-5214-4277-9

定价 **39.00 元**

获取新书信息、投稿、为图书纠错，请扫码联系我们。

前　言

　　本教材传承上版教材的主要特色，共包括净制、切制、炒法、炙法、煅法、蒸法、燀法、其他方法和设计性实验等23个实验。每个实验内容包括实验目的、实验原理、实验器材、实验内容和实验指导等5个模块。通过5个模块的学习和训练，使学生掌握中药炮制基本的操作方法和技能，更好地理解中药炮制的目的及意义。本版在内容上增加了传统炮制方法中的炒、炙、煅、蒸、煮、燀及其他方法等代表药物的炮制内容，删减了个别实验结果难以重复的实验，内容紧密结合《中国药典》，更新了实验内容，体现了传统与现代结合的特点。本教材为双语教材，通过双语的形式，使更多的非汉语学生了解中药炮制学，同时使汉语学生专业英语水平有所提高。本教材适用于全日制中药学、中药资源与开发、中药制药学、药学等相关专业师生教学使用，亦可作为医药院校、职业院校药学专业或医药人员及中药炮制实验技术人员参考资料。

　　在本教材编写过程中，得到了中药炮制界同仁、各编写单位的鼎力支持和热心帮助，在此一并致以深深的谢意。鉴于编者学识所限，本教材难免存在疏漏、不妥之处，恳请广大读者批评和指正。

编　者

2023 年 10 月

目 录

·•· 第四章 煅法 ·•·

·•· 第五章 蒸法 ·•·

·•· 第六章 煮法 ·•·

·•· 第七章 焯法 ·•·

·•· 第八章 其他制法 ·•·

·•· 第九章 设计性实验 ·•·

第一章　净制、切制

实验一　净制、切制

实验目的 ●●

1. 掌握药材的净制方法、基本要求以及软化方法、软化程度及软化条件。
2. 掌握手工切制、机器切制及饮片干燥的方法。
3. 熟悉常见的饮片类型及规格。
4. 了解净制和切制的目的。

实验原理 ●●

中药材来源于动物、植物的不同部位，在采收、贮存和运输过程中，常会带入杂质。去除杂质和非药用部位，以提高有效成分相对含量，保证用量准确，从而保证临床药效。

干燥的药材细胞皱缩，不便切制，需要软化。而动植物药材几乎都含蛋白质、淀粉、纤维素等亲水性物质，是药材能够被水软化的必要条件。将药材用水清洗浸润，表面先湿润、吸水，从而在药材表面与中心之间形成湿度差，水分逐渐向中心部位渗透使药材软化。药材被软化的过程除了与其体形大小有关，还与药材的组织结构、水温等有关。

气相置换法软化药材的基本原理：将装有药材的密闭箱体抽成真空状态，药材内部空隙也成真空状态，当有水蒸气注入时，水蒸气进入药材内部的空隙，药材的亲水物质吸水膨胀而逐渐软化。在软化过程中，药材内部空隙的压力小于外部水蒸气的压力，外部水蒸气就会不断地补充这些空隙，直至水分饱和，药材软化。该法可缩短软化时间，提高软化效率。

实验器材 ●●

1. **仪器**　蒸煮容器，搪瓷盘，切药刀，刷子，旋转式切药机，往复式切药机，真空置换润药机，电热恒温干燥箱等。

2. **药材**　党参，牛膝，陈皮，枇杷叶，黄芩，淫羊藿，川芎，金樱子等。

实验内容 ●●

1. 净制

（1）党参、牛膝　切去芦头，抢水洗。

（2）陈皮　挑选，去除果柄，发霉变质品、伪品等，抢水洗。

（3）枇杷叶　用毛刷去除绒毛，抢水洗。

（4）黄芩　去除茎残基。

（5）淫羊藿　除去杂质，摘取叶片。

（6）川芎　除去杂质，大小分档，抢水洗。

（7）金樱子　除去杂质，洗净略浸，润透，纵切两瓣，除去毛、核。

2. 软化

（1）冷浸软化

党参、牛膝　分别将抢水冲洗后的净党参、净牛膝，置搪瓷盘中排放整齐，以湿布覆盖，不时喷洒适量清水，润至弯曲法检查合格。

陈皮　将洗净陈皮铺在瓷盘内，湿纱布覆盖，不时喷洒适量清水，闷润至湿度均匀、内外一致。

枇杷叶　将净枇杷叶抢水洗，稍润。

淫羊藿　将净淫羊藿抢水洗，稍润。

（2）加热软化

黄芩　取净黄芩，大小分档，置蒸制容器内隔水加热，蒸至圆汽后半小时，至质地软化，内外一致，取出趁热切片。

（3）真空软化

川芎　将净川芎置于真空置换润药机内，按操作规程操作，至软化适度。

3. 切制

（1）手工切制

切药刀切制　先固定切药刀，将药材放置在刀床上，根据切制饮片厚度，选择软硬不同的木制压板，左手掌握压板，压紧药材，右手持刀，两手配合切片。

片刀切制　一手拿软化好的药物，一手拿切刀，两手配合，切片。

（2）机器切制　首先检查机器各部件，然后试机，再根据各药选择适宜的片型、厚度进行调节和固定刀口的位置，即可切片。

（3）规格要求

党参、川芎（蝴蝶片）切为2～4 mm的厚片。

黄芩切为2～4 mm的斜片。

陈皮切为2～3 mm的细丝。

枇杷叶（顺一侧叶脉方向切制）、淫羊藿切为5～10 mm的宽丝。

牛膝切为4～8 mm段。

4. 干燥

（1）自然干燥　将切制后的饮片置于竹匾或其他容器内阴干、风干或晒干。干燥过程中定时翻动，以达到充分干燥（黄芩片避免暴晒）。

（2）人工干燥　将切制后的饮片置于钢网筛或适宜容器内，放入烘箱，根据药品饮片性质，分别控制适宜温度和时间，定时翻动至全部干燥，取出放凉。

实验指导 ●●●

1. 基本操作和操作注意点

（1）浸润软化时水分要适当，坚持"少泡多润，药透水尽"的基本原则。软化"太过"或"不及"均影响饮片质量或增加切制难度。

（2）机器切制要注意随时检查机器，按章操作，杜绝事故。

（3）手工切制要注意掌握压板向前移动速度，持刀从旁持握，放刀平稳。

（4）陈皮饮片干燥时，因陈皮含挥发油类成分，干燥温度不超过50℃。

2. 实验报告格式

（1）实验目的

（2）实验原理

（3）实验内容

（4）讨论

3. 实验后思考

（1）药材为什么要切制成饮片？

（2）药材浸泡对药材质量和切制有何影响？

（3）饮片干燥时为什么要控制适宜温度？

（李　凯　孙小雅）

Experiment 1　Cleansing and Cutting Procedure

◆ Experimental purposes

1. To master the methods and basic requirements for cleansing, as well as the method, degree and conditions of softening.

2. To familarize the methods of manual cutting, machine cutting and drying the decoction pieces.

3. To understand the types and specifications of the common decoction pieces.

4. To know the purposes of cleansing and cutting procedure.

◆ Experimental principle

Chinese medicinal materials are derived from the different parts of natural plants and animals. Some impurities are often brought in during the procedures of collection, storage and transportation. To increase the contents of effective components and ensure accurate medicinal dosage, the impurities and non-medicinal parts are needed to be removed.

Cells of dried drug are always shrunken, which leads to cut difficultly, so the dried drug should be softened before cutting. Natural plants and animals contain hydrophilic components, the necessities of medicinal softening, such as protein, starch and cellulose. Firstly, the drug is infiltrated in water and the hygrometric deficits are formed between the surface and center of the drug. Subsequently, the water will gradually infiltrate towards the center areas of the drug until it is softened. The softening procedure is related to many factors including the size of the drug, organization structures and water temperature.

The fundamental of gas phase displacement to soften drug: when closed chamber containing the drug is vacuumized, the pores inside the drug are in vacuum. With the injection of vapor, the streams enter the pores inside the herb. Then, the hydrophilic substances in the herb absorb water and swell, which results in softening of herb gradually. During the softening process, the pressure inside the drug is less than that of the vapor outside. Thus, streams outside the drug will fill the pores continuously until the water is saturated and the drug softened. This method can shorten the softening time and improve its efficiency.

◆ Experimental apparatus

1. Instruments

Cooking container, enameled dish, cutting knife, brush, rotary cutter machine, reciprocating cutter machine, vacuum permutation embellish medicine machine, electrothermal constant-temperature dry box.

2. Medicinal materials

Codonopsis Radix, Achyranthis Bidentatae Radix, Citri Reticulatae Pericarpium, Eriobotryae Folium, Scutellariae Radix, Epimedii Folium, Chuanxiong Rhizoma, Rosae Laevigatae Fructus.

◆ Experimental content

1. Cleansing

1.1 Codonopsis Radix, Achyranthis Bidentatae Radix: Cut off the basal part of stem and wash quickly.

1.2 Citri Reticulatae Pericarpium: Select and remove the fruit stalks, mouldy drugs and counterfeits, and wash quickly.

1.3 Eriobotryae Folium: Remove villus with brush and wash quickly.

1.4 Scutellariae Radix: Remove stem residues.

1.5 Epimedii Folium: Remove impurities and pick leaves.

1.6 Chuanxiong Rhizoma: Remove impurities, size grading, and wash quickly.

1.7 Rosae Laevigatae Fructus: Remove impurities, wash and dip, cut the drug longitudinally into two parts and remove hair and core.

2. Softening

2.1 Softening with cold water

Codonopsis Radix and Achyranthis Bidentatae Radix: Place the quickly washed Codonopsis Radix and Achyranthis Bidentatae Radix on enameled dish orderly, cover with a wet cloth, and then spray water irregularly. Check the softening degree with bending method.

Citri Reticulatae Pericarpium: Place clean Citri Reticulatae Pericarpium on an enameled dish orderly, cover with a wet cloth, and spray water irregularly until the humidity inside is similar to the outside.

Eriobotryae Folium: Wash Eriobotryae Folium quickly and dip slightly.

Epimedii Folium: Wash Epimedii Folium quickly and dip slightly.

2.2 Softening with heating

Scutellariae Radix: Separate the different sizes of clean Scutellariae Radix. Put them into a cooking container and heat over simmering water for 30 minutes until the drugs are softened to the similar extent thoroughly. Then cut them quickly.

2.3 Softening with vacuum

Chuanxiong Rhizoma: Put clean Chuanxiong Rhizoma into a vacuum permutation embellish medicine machine and operate according to the specifications till the drug is softened moderately.

3. Cutting

3.1 Manual cutting

Cutting by the cutting knife: First, fix the cutting knife and place the drug on the cutting and select wooden pressing-plates with different hardness according to the thickness of the slices. Fix the drug with the prtessing-plate by one hand and take the cutting knife in another hand to cut.

Cutting by a slice knife: Fix the softened drug with one hand and hold the slice knife in another hand to cut.

3.2 Cutting by machine

First, check the machine and pilot run. Then, adjust and fix the knife edge according to the thickness and types of the slices to cut.

3.3 Specification requirements

Codonopsis Radix and Chuanxiong Rhizoma: Cut into thick slices of 2-4 mm.

Scutellariae Radix：Cut into oblique slices of 2-4 mm.

Citri Reticulatae Pericarpium：Cut into threadlets of 2-3 mm.

Eriobotryae Folium and Epimedii Folium：Cut into wide filaments of 5-10 mm.

Achyranthis Bidentatae Radix：Cut into sections of 4-8 mm.

4. Drying

4.1 Natural drying

Place the decoction pieces in a bamboo basket or other containers in the shadow, air or sun, and stir at fixed intervals to ensure them to be dried completely.

4.2 Drying in oven

Place the decoction pieces in steel mesh sieve or container in oven, and stir at fixed intervals to ensure them to be dried completely. The temperature and period should be controlled according to the characteristics of the herb. Then take them out and cool.

◆ Experimental instruction

1. Primary operation and the notes of the operation

1.1 During the procedure of infiltration, drugs should be infiltrated more and soaked less to make them infiltrate thoroughly and the water be absorbed entirely. The softening degree will both influence the quality of slices and cutting process.

1.2 Check the machine anytime when automatic cutting. Operate according to the operation specifications.

1.3 The moving speed of pressing-plate should be controlled and the cutter should be taken from edgeways and put down stably.

1.4 When the slices of Citri Reticulatae Pericarpium are dried, the temperature should not be higher than 50℃ because of their volatile components.

2. Format of the experimental report

2.1 Purposes

2.2 Principle

2.3 The content of the experiment

2.4 Discussion

3. Considerations after the experiment

3.1 Why should the crude drug be cut into slices?

3.2 What is the impact of soaking on the herbal quality and cutting procedure?

3.3 Why should the temperature be controlled at a suitable level when drying the slices?

(Edited by Kai Li and Xiaoya Sun)

第二章　炒　法

实验二　炒法代表药物炮制

实验目的 •••

1. 掌握炒黄、炒焦、炒炭、麸炒、砂炒、土炒、米炒、蛤粉炒的基本操作方法、注意事项及饮片质量要求。

2. 掌握清炒法的不同火候，炒后药性的变化及炒炭"存性"的含义。

3. 掌握麸炒、砂炒、土炒、米炒、蛤粉炒的火候控制及注意事项。

4. 了解清炒和加固体辅料炒的目的和意义。

实验原理 •••

炒法分为清炒和加辅料炒两种。清炒包括炒黄、炒焦、炒炭。根据辅料的不同，加辅料炒分为麸炒、砂炒、土炒、米炒、蛤粉炒、滑石粉炒。炒制的目的是为了缓和药性，增强疗效，降低毒性或副作用，增强或产生止血作用，保存疗效利于贮存等。

炒黄的药物大部分为种子类药物，种皮坚实，难以粉碎，有效成分不易煎出。炒黄可使种皮爆裂，组织疏松，便于粉碎，利于有效成分的煎出和调剂；炒焦可以缓和药性，增加健脾和中功效，有"焦香醒脾"之说；炒炭可使药物产生或增强止血作用，有"炒炭止血"之说。

固体辅料具有中间传热体的作用，能使药物受热均匀，炒后的饮片色泽一致，外观质量好，质地酥脆，易于粉碎，有效成分易于煎出，利于调剂和制剂。砂炒及滑石粉炒因火力强，温度高，适于炒制质地坚硬或韧性大的动物类药物。此外，砂炒及滑石粉炒可使某些药物的毒性成分结构改变或破坏，从而降低其毒性。米与药物同炒，一方面米能吸附某些昆虫类药物的毒性成分，另一方面，加热也能使毒性成分破坏，从而降低药物的毒性。蛤粉炒由于火力较弱，且蛤粉颗粒细小，传热作用较慢，使药物缓慢均匀受热，适于炒制胶类药物。

实验器材 •••

1. 仪器　炒锅，锅铲，电磁炉，瓷盘，筛子，温度计，天平，喷壶等。

2. 药材

（1）炒黄　槐米、莱菔子、王不留行、冬瓜子。

（2）炒焦　山楂、栀子。

（3）炒炭　蒲黄、荆芥、槐米。

（4）麸炒　苍术、枳壳、麦麸。

（5）砂炒　粗河砂、鸡内金、骨碎补。

（6）土炒　灶心土、山药、白术。

（7）米炒　大米、党参。

（8）蛤粉炒　蛤粉、阿胶。

实验内容 •••

1. 炒黄 e 微课1

（1）炒槐米　取净槐米，置热锅内，用文火炒至表面深黄色，取出，摊凉。

（2）炒莱菔子　取净莱菔子，置热锅内，用文火炒至微鼓起，有密集爆裂声，手捻易碎，种仁黄色，富油性，有香气时，取出摊凉。

（3）炒王不留行　取净王不留行，置热锅内，用中火炒至大多数爆白花，取出，晾凉。

（4）炒冬瓜子　取净冬瓜子，置热锅内，用文火炒至表面略黄色，稍有焦斑，取出，摊凉。

2. 炒焦 e 微课2

（1）焦山楂　取净山楂，置热锅内，用中火炒至表面焦褐色，内部焦黄色，取出摊晾，筛去灰屑和脱落的果核。

（2）焦栀子　取净栀子碎块，置热锅内，用文火炒至黄褐色，取出，摊晾。

3. 炒炭 e 微课3

（1）蒲黄炭　取净蒲黄，置热锅内，中火加热，不断翻炒至焦褐色，若有火星，喷淋少量清水熄灭，略炒干，取出，晾干。

（2）荆芥炭　取净荆芥段，置热锅内，武火加热，不断翻炒至黑褐色，若有火星，喷淋少许清水熄灭，略炒干，取出，晾干，筛去灰屑。

（3）槐米炭　取净槐米，置热锅内，中火加热，不断翻炒至黑褐色，若有火星，喷淋少许清水熄灭，炒干，取出放凉，筛去灰屑。

4. 麸炒 e 微课4

（1）苍术　先将麦麸撒于热锅内，中火加热，冒烟时投入适量苍术片，翻炒至表面深黄色，取出。筛去麦麸，放凉。每100kg苍术片，用麦麸10kg。

（2）枳壳　先将麦麸撒于热锅内，中火加热，冒烟时投入适量枳壳片，迅速翻动，炒至枳壳表面深黄色时，取出。筛去麦麸，放凉。每100kg枳壳片，用麦麸10kg。

5. 砂炒

（1）鸡内金　取河砂置热锅内，中火加热至滑利时，投入鸡内金，翻炒至鼓起、酥脆，呈淡黄色时取出，筛去砂，摊晾。

（2）骨碎补　取河砂置热锅内，武火加热至滑利时，投入骨碎补片，翻炒至鼓起，取出，筛去砂，撞去毛，摊晾。

6. 土炒 e 微课5

（1）山药　将灶心土粉置热锅内，中火加热至土呈灵活状态，投入山药片拌炒，至表面均匀挂土粉、药透香气时取出，筛去土粉，摊晾。每100kg山药饮片，用灶心土粉30kg。

（2）白术　将灶心土粉置热锅内，中火加热至土呈灵活状态时，投入白术片拌炒，至表面均匀挂土色，药透香气时取出，筛去土粉，摊晾。每100kg白术片，用灶心土粉20kg。

7. 米炒 e 微课6

米炒党参　将米置热锅内，用中火加热至冒烟时，投入党参片拌炒，至党参表面深黄色，米呈焦黄或焦褐色时取出，筛去米，摊晾。每100kg党参片，用米20kg。

8. 蛤粉炒

蛤粉炒阿胶　取蛤粉置热锅内，用中火加热至灵活状态时，投入阿胶丁，不断翻动，炒至鼓起呈圆球形，内部呈蜂窝状，无溏心，质松泡时，取出，筛去蛤粉，摊晾。每100kg药物，用蛤粉30~50kg。

实验指导 ●●●

1. 预习

（1）砂炒鸡内金、骨碎补的炮制原理是什么？土炒山药、白术的炮制原理是什么？米炒党参的炮制原理是什么？蛤粉炒阿胶的炮制原理是什么？

（2）中药炮制"去毛"的方法有哪些？为什么去毛？

（3）党参为何要炮制？炮制方法有哪些？

（4）阿胶为何要炮制？方法有哪些？

（5）加辅料炒制的温度对药物有什么影响？

（6）什么是火候？在炒制操作中如何把握？

2. 基本操作和操作注意点

（1）炒前药物应净选除杂，大小分档。炒制时选择适当火力，并控制炮制时间。质地坚实者宜用武火，质地疏松者可用中火。

（2）操作时，先预热锅，勤翻动，使药物受热均匀，避免生熟不匀的现象。

（3）炒黄需防止焦化；炒焦需防止炭化；炒炭需防止灰化。

（4）炒炭要注意防火，炒制过程中出现火星应及时喷洒少量清水熄灭。取出后必须摊开放凉，检查无复燃再收存。

（5）每种饮片火候各有侧重，应注意区别，如炒槐米、炒冬瓜子、焦山楂、焦栀子等以颜色为主要判断依据，炒莱菔子以爆裂声为主要判断依据，炒王不留行以爆花率为判断依据。

（6）炒制王不留行时，为避免生熟不均，每次投药量应少，宜用毛刷或炊帚作为翻动工具，翻动频率也应先慢后快。

（7）麸炒药物火力可稍大，麦麸要均匀撒布热锅中，待起烟后投药。借麸皮之烟熏使药物变色，但火力过大，则麸皮迅速焦黑，达不到麸炒的目的。

（8）砂炒温度应适中，砂的用量以能掩盖所加药物为度，以保证受热均匀；砂的温度过高时可以通过添加冷砂或减小火力等方法加以调节。

（9）灶心土呈灵活状态时投入山药后，要适当调小火力，维持土温，防止烫焦；用土炒同种药物时，灶心土可重复使用，若土色变深时，应及时换新土。

（10）炮制达到火候后要迅速出锅，出锅后迅速摊开晾凉，避免炮制过度。

（11）米炒时可以以米的色泽判断火候，拌炒至米呈焦黄或焦褐色可作为判断炮制火候的标准之一。

（12）先将胶块切成大小适合的立方丁，大小分档后，分别炒制。炒制时，翻炒速度要快而均匀，否则会引起互相粘连，造成不圆整而影响外观。尤其要注意控制温度，一般蛤粉温度在180℃左右，温度高于200℃易炭化，低于160℃不易鼓起，且表面粗糙。

3. 实验报告格式

（1）实验目的

（2）实验原理

（3）实验内容

（4）讨论

4. 实验后思考

（1）炒炭存性的含义和意义？

（2）火候的判断标准是什么？

（3）炒炭多用"武火"，为什么蒲黄和槐米炒炭要用"中火"？

（4）炒王不留行的炮制目的及注意事项是什么？

（5）炒焦栀子时，为何先将栀子碾碎？

（6）除传统土炒和麸炒外，还可采用哪些现代工艺炮制山药，现代技术与传统技术相比有何优势和不足？山药经炮制后，其药理性质发生哪些变化？

（7）采用哪些检测指标和方法用于研究炮制对鸡内金有效成分的影响？

（8）根据文献说明哪些现代技术可以用于改进骨碎补的炮制？

（9）阿胶的炮制方法有哪些？分析阿胶炮制的目的是什么？

（10）加固体辅料炒法中不同的辅料各起什么作用？

（11）为什么要严格控制辅料的用量？

（李　凯　张春凤　李　飞）

书网融合……

微课1　　　　微课2　　　　微课3　　　　微课4　　　　微课5　　　　微课6

Experiment 2　Representative Drug Processed by Stir-frying

◆ Experimental purposes

1. To familiarize the basic processing methods, precautions and quality requirements of stir-frying drug to yellow, brown and charcoal; stir-frying with bran, sand, oven earth, rice, and pulverized-clamshell.

2. To master the heating degree of stir-frying drug to yellow, brown and charcoal; and to understand the changes in medicinal properties after stir-frying drug and the meaning of preserving the nature of the herb after stir-frying drug to charcoal.

3. To learn about the heating degree and precautions of stir-frying with bran, sand, oven earth, rice, and pulverized-clamshell.

4. To understand the processing purpose and significance of stir-frying drug with and without solid adjuvant.

◆ Experimental principle

The processing methods of stir-frying drugs in a caldron include stir-frying drug with and without solid adjuvant. The processing methods of stir-frying drug without adjuvant include stir-frying drug to yellow, brown and charcoal. Usually, stir-frying drug to yellow needs mild heating fire, stir-frying drug to brown over medium heat, and stir-frying drug to charcoal with strong fire. According to different adjuvant used, the processing methods of stir-frying drug with solid adjuvant include stir-frying with bran, sand, oven earth, rice, pulverized-clamshell and pulverized-talcum. The purpose of stir-frying drug is to moderate the medicinal properties, enhance the therapeutic effects, reduce toxicity or side effects, enhance or produce hemostatic effect and preserve the therapeutic effects for storage, etc.

Most of the stir-frying drug to yellow are seeds. The seed coat is solid and difficult to crush, so the active ingredients are not easy to be decocted. Stir-frying drug to yellow can make the seed coat burst, loosen the tissue, facilitate the crushing, the decoction of the active ingredients and further conditioning, etc. There is the experience that the seed drugs must be stir-frying before using in the processing. Stir-frying drug to brown can moderate the medicinal properties and increase the efficacy of strengthening the spleen and harmonizing the middle, so there is the theory of caramelized aroma to awaken the spleen in the processing. Stir-frying drug to charcoal can produce or enhance the effect of stopping bleeding, and there is a doctrine that blood stops when it meets black. Stir-frying drug can be better adapted to clinical needs and improve the target of treatment and safety of medication.

Solid adjuvant has the role of intermediate heat transfer body, which can make the drug heated evenly. The drug of stir-frying with solid adjuvant has the same color and luster, good quality appearance, crispy texture, easy to crush and decoct out the active ingredients, which is convenient for transferring and preparation. Stir-frying with sand and with pulverized-talcum is suitable for hard texture or toughness of animal drug because of the stronger fire and higher temperature. In addition, they can reduce the toxicity of certain drug by changing or destroying the structure of their toxic components. As for stir-frying drug with rice, on the one hand, rice can adsorb the toxic components of certain insect drug, on the other hand, heating can also destroy the toxic components, so it can reduce the toxicity of drug. Stir-frying with pulverized-clamshell is suitable for stir-frying drug like Asini Corii Colla because it requires low heat, the particles of clam powder are fine and the heat transfer is slow, which can make the drug heated slowly and evenly.

◆ Experimental apparatus

1. Instruments

Pot, spatula, induction cooker, porcelain plate, sieve, thermometer, balance, spray bottle, etc.

2. Medicinal materials

2.1 Stir-frying drug to yellow: Sophorae Flos, Raphani Semen, Vaccariae Semen, wax gourd seeds.

2.2 Stir-frying drug to brown: Crataegi Fructus, Gardeniae Fructus.

2.3 Stir-frying drug to charcoal: Typhae Pollen, Schizonepetae Herba, and Sophorae Flos.

2.4 Stir-frying with wheat bran: Atractylodis Rhizoma, Aurantii Fructus, and wheat bran.

2.5 Stir-frying with sand: Galli Gigeriae Endothelium Corneum, Drynariae Rhizoma, and coarse river sand.

2.6 Stir-frying with oven earth: Dioscoreae Rhizoma, Atractylodis Macrocephalae Rhizoma, and oven earth.

2.7 Stir-frying with rice: Codonopsis Rhizoma, and rice.

2.8 Stir-frying with pulverized-clamshell: Asini Corii Colla, and pulverized-clamshell.

◆ Experimental content

1. Stir-frying drug to yellow

1.1 Sophorae Flos (Huaimi)

Put clean Flos Sophorae in a moderately preheated frying container and stir fry until the surface is dark yellow. Chill before serving.

1.2 Raphani Semen (Laifuzi)

Put clean Semen Raphani in a moderately preheated frying container and stir fry until slightly swollen, with a dense popping sound and fragility. The seeds are yellow and oily. Chill before serving. Mash before using.

1.3 Vaccariae Semen (Wangbuliuxing)

Take clean Vaccariae Semen, place them in a moderately preheated frying container and stir fry until most of the white flowers appear. Chill before serving.

1.4 Wax gourd seeds (Dongguazi)

Take clean wax gourd seeds, place them in a moderately preheated frying container and stir fry until the surface is slightly yellow and a small amount of burned dots appear. Chill before serving.

2. Stir-frying drug to brown

2.1 Crataegi Fructus (Shanzha)

Put clean Crataegi Fructus in a moderately preheated frying container and stir fry until the surface is burnt brown and the inside becomes yellow. Chill before serving. Sieve off dust and dropped fruit kernels.

2.2 Gardeniae Fructus (Zhizi)

Put clean broken pieces of Gardeniae Fructus in a moderately preheated frying container and stir fry until golden brown. Chill before serving.

3. Stir-frying drug to charcoal

3.1 Typhae Pollen (Puhuang)

Put an appropriate amount of the clean Typhae Pollen in a hot pot, heat over medium heat, and stir constantly until becoming brown. If there is a spark, spray a small amount of water to extinguish, and slightly stir-fry dry.

3.2 Schizonepetae Herba (Jingjie)

Put an appropriate amount of the clean Schizonepetae Herba in a hot pot, heat with strong heating fire, stir constantly until becoming focal brown. If there is a spark, spray a small amount of water to extinguish, slightly stir-fry dry.

3.3 Sophorae Flos (Huaimi)

Put an appropriate amount of the clean Sophorae Flos in a hot pot, heat over medium heat, stir constantly until becoming focal brown. If there is a spark, spray a small amount of water to extinguish, stir-fry dry and sieve off the ash chips after cooling.

4. Stir-frying with wheat bran

4.1 Atractylodis Rhizoma (Cangzhu)

Atractylodis Rhizoma stir-fried with wheat bran: Spread wheat bran into the hot pot evenly. Put the clean Atractylodis Rhizoma slices in the pot while smoking. Stir-frying over medium heat until becoming dark yellow. Sift out wheat bran. Chill before serving. For every 100kg of Atractylodis Rhizoma, use 10kg of wheat bran.

4.2 Aurantii Fructus (Zhiqiao)

Aurantii Fructus stir-fried with wheat bran: Spread wheat bran into the hot pot evenly. Put the clean Aurantii Fructus slices in the pot while smoking. Stir-frying over medium heat until becoming pale yellow. Chill before serving, and then sift out wheat bran. For every 100kg of Aurantii Fructus, use 10kg of wheat bran.

5. Stir-frying with sand

5.1 Galli Gigeriae Endothelium Corneum (Jineijing)

Put the river sand in a moderately preheated frying container. When the sand becomes smooth, put in the chicken gold, stir fry until swollen and crisp, and take it out when being dark yellow. Sieve to remove the sand. Chill before serving.

5.2 Drynariae Rhizoma (Gusuibu)

Put the river sand in a moderately preheated frying container. When the sand becomes smooth, put the drug in the pot, stir fry until being swollen, remove hair and sand. Chill before serving.

6. Stir-frying with oven earth

6.1 Dioscoreae Rhizoma (Shanyao)

Put the oven earth in the pre-heated frying container until soft, add the Dioscoreae Rhizoma to stir fry, and remove it when the surface is evenly hung with the soil powder and fragrant. Sieve the soil powder. Chill before serving. For every 100kg of Dioscoreae Rhizoma, 30kg of oven earth will be used.

6.2 Atractylodis Macrocephalae Rhizoma (Baizhu)

Put the oven earth in a preheated frying container, heat until soft, add Atractylodis Macrocephalae Rhizoma and stir fry until the surface is evenly covered with earth color and fragrant, remove the soil powder. Chill before serving. For every 100kg Atractylodis Macrocephalae Rhizoma, use 20kg oven earth.

7. Stir-frying with rice

Codonopsis Rhizoma（Dangshen）

Put the rice in a preheated frying container, heat it to smoke, stir fry the Codonopsis Rhizoma slices, until the drug surface is dark yellow, the rice is scorched yellow or scorched brown, sieve the rice. Chill before serving. For every 100kg of Codonopsis Rhizoma tablets, 20kg of rice will be used.

8. Stir-frying with pulverized-clamshell

Asini Corii Colla（Ejiao）

Put appropriate amount of clam powder in a preheated frying container. When it is stir-fried with medium heat to a flexible state, add Asini Corii Colla tin and stir it constantly. When the clam powder is bulging and spherical, the inside is honeycomb-like, and the quality is loose and bubbly instead of runny, sieve the clam powder. Chill before serving. For every 100kg of medication, 30 to 50kg of clam powder will be used.

◆ Experiment instruction

1. Preview

1.1 How do you think the processing principle of Galli Gigeriae Endothelium Corneum, Drynariae Rhizoma, Dioscoreae Rhizoma, Atractylodis Macrocephalae Rhizoma, Codonopsis Rhizoma and Asini Corii Colla?

1.2 How many are the methods of "removing hair" there and why?

1.3 Why does the Codonopsis Rhizoma need to process? What methods?

1.4 Why does the Asini Corii Colla need to process? What methods?

1.5 How does the temperature of stir-frying drug with solid adjuvant affect the drug?

1.6 How to grasp the heat in the operation of stir-frying drug?

2. Primary operation and the notes of the operation

2.1 Separate the crude by size before stir-frying. Choose the proper temperature when stir-frying and control the heating time. Firm-textured drug should be processed with strong fire while loose-textured drug over medium heat.

2.2 Preheat the pot first before stir-frying and stir frequently to heat the drug evenly.

2.3 Prevent scorching during stir-frying drug to yellow, carbonization during brown, and ashing during charcoal.

2.4 Pay attention to fire protection during stir-frying drug to charcoal. If a spark is found, please spray some water to extinguish in time. No reburning before storing.

2.5 Pay attention to different crude slices' emphasis on heat. For example, Flos Sophorae, wax gourd seeds, Charred Crataegi Fructus and Charred Gardeniae Fructus, during stir frying, color as main criterion for judgment, for Semen Raphani, popping sound as criterion, while for Vaccariae Semen, popping percentage is for judgment.

2.6 As for Vaccariae Semen, to avoid uneven ripeness, the coagulant dosage should be small each time. It is advisable to use a brush or cooking brush as the flipping tool, and the flipping frequency should also be slow first and then fast.

2.7 As for stir-frying with bran, the fire should be slightly stronger. Wheat bran is evenly spread in the hot pot, and put the clean drug in the pot while smoking. The smoke of the wheat bran is used to discolor the drug, and no strong fire needed, otherwise, the wheat bran quickly scorched black and no purpose of stir-frying with bran achieved.

2.8 The temperature of sand fry is moderate, and the amount of sand can cover the medicine to ensure uniform heating; When the temperature is too high, it can be adjusted by adding cold sand or reducing the heat.

2.9 When the soil is in a flexible state, the Dioscoreae Rhizoma is put into the stove, and then the fire should be appropriately reduced to maintain the temperature of the soil and to prevent scorching; When frying the same kind of medicine with soil, the soil can be used continuously. If the soil color becomes dark, new soil should be replaced in time.

2.10 After processing, products should be taken out of the pot quickly to avoid excessive processing.

2.11 When frying, the rice color can be observed in the heat until yellow or brown, as one of the criteria for judging the processing heat.

2.12 First cut the glue block into cubes of suitable size, respectively fried. When frying, the speed should be fast and uniform, otherwise it will cause adhesion, resulting in non-roundness and affect the appearance. In particular, it is needed to pay attention to the control of the temperature. The temperature of the clam powder is about 180℃, and it is easy to char when higher than 200℃, and the surface is rough but not easy to bulge when lower than 160℃.

3. Format of the experimental report

3.1 Purposes

3.2 Principle

3.3 The content of the experiment

3.4 Discussion

4. Considerations after the experiment

4.1 How to understand the meaning of preserving the nature of the drug after stir-frying drug to charcoal?

4.2 What are the criteria for judging the heating degree?

4.3 Usually, stir-frying drug to charcoal needs strong heating fire, but stir-frying Typhae Pollen and Sophorae Flos to charcoal need medium heating. How to explain it?

4.4 Briefly describe the purposes and precautions of stir-frying Vaccariae Semen.

4.5 Why grind the Gardeniae Fructus first when stir-frying them to brown?

4.6 In addition to the traditional stir-frying with soil and bran, what other modern techniques can process Dioscoreae Rhizoma, and what are the advantages and disadvantages of modern technology compared with traditional one? How does the pharmacological property of Dioscoreae Rhizoma change after processing?

4.7 What are the detection indicators and methods to compare the effect of processing on the effective ingredients of Galli Gigeriae Endothelium Corneum?

4.8 According to the literature reviewed, what other modern techniques can improve the processing of Drynariae Rhizoma?

4.9 What are the processing methods of Asini Corii Colla and what are the effects? What is the purpose of analyzing the processing of Asini Corii Colla?

4.10 What is the role of different solid adjuvants in stir-frying with solid adjuvant?

4.11 Why is it necessary to strictly control the amount of solid adjuvant?

(Edited by Kai Li, Chunfeng Zhang and Fei Li)

实验三　槐米及其炮制品中芦丁、鞣质的含量测定

实验目的 ●●●

1. 掌握芦丁、鞣质的含量测定方法。

2. 通过对槐米炮制前后芦丁和鞣质含量的比较，了解炮制槐米的作用和意义。

实验原理 ●●●

槐米为豆科植物槐 *Sophora japonica* L. 的干燥花蕾，为凉血、止血药，用于便血、痔血、血痢、崩漏、吐血、衄血等。槐米中含有芦丁和少量的三萜皂苷，后者水解后得到白桦脂醇、槐二醇、葡萄糖、葡萄糖醛酸；另含有鞣质。其中鞣质具有收敛、固涩、止血、止痢以及抗菌消炎的作用。

传统经验认为，槐米炒炭后能缓和其寒性，产生涩性，从而增强止血作用；现代研究证实槐米炒炭后鞣质含量增加，止血作用明显增强。

本实验采用高效液相色谱法以及高锰酸钾法或干酪素法分别测定槐米中芦丁和鞣质的含量。

实验器材 ●●●

1. 仪器　高效液相色谱仪，C$_{18}$色谱柱，100mL具塞锥形瓶，超声波提取器，紫外分光光度计，分析天平，10mL刻度吸管、10mL、25mL、100mL、500mL量瓶，10mL、50mL棕色量瓶，100mL圆底烧瓶，10mL、500mL量筒，棕色贮液瓶，10mL、25mL酸式滴定管，乳钵，真空干燥箱，烧杯，移液管，垂熔玻璃漏斗，分液漏斗，滤纸，索氏提取器，水浴锅，电炉，震荡器，冷凝管，温度计（300℃），玻棒等。

2. 药材及试剂　槐米，槐米炮制品，芦丁对照品，KMnO$_4$，靛胭脂，浓硫酸，氯化钠，硫酸钡，明胶，碳酸钠，钨酸，磷酸，冰醋酸（CR），甲醇（CR、AR）。

实验内容 ●●●

1. 芦丁的含量测定

（1）色谱条件　以十八烷基硅烷键合硅胶为填充剂；以甲醇–1%冰醋酸溶液（32∶68）为流动相；检测波长为257nm。

（2）对照品溶液的制备　取芦丁对照品适量，精密称定，加甲醇制成每1mL含0.1mg的溶液，即得。

（3）供试品溶液的制备　取本品粗粉约0.1g，精密称定，置具塞锥形瓶中，精密加入甲醇50mL，称定重量，超声处理（功率250W，频率25kHz）30分钟，放冷，再称定重量，用甲醇补足减失的重量，摇匀，滤过。精密量取续滤液2mL，置10mL量瓶中，加甲醇至刻度，摇匀，即得。

（4）测定方法　分别精密吸取对照品溶液与供试品溶液各10μL，注入液相色谱仪，测定，即得。

2. 鞣质的含量测定

（1）高锰酸钾法

① 分别取槐米和槐米炭粗粉，约10g，精密称定，加水300mL，小火煮沸30分钟，滤过。药渣再加水100mL重复提取2次，滤过，合并3次滤液，定容于500mL量瓶中，静置过夜。次日过滤，精密吸取续滤液10mL于1000mL锥形瓶中，加500mL水、5mL 0.6%的靛胭脂、20mL硫酸，用0.02 mol/L

KMnO$_4$溶液滴定至出现黄绿色，消耗KMnO$_4$溶液的毫升数记为"A"。

② 空白溶液的测定：精密吸取上述提取液100mL，加入30mL新鲜配制的明胶溶液，用氯化钠饱和，加10mL 10%的稀硫酸及10g硫酸钡，振摇数分钟，滤过。吸取滤液10mL，同上法用0.02mol/L KMnO$_4$溶液滴定，消耗KMnO$_4$溶液的毫升数记为"B"。

③ 槐米中鞣质含量的计算：以鞣酸为标准，每1mL 0.1 mol/L KMnO$_4$溶液相当于0.004157g鞣酸。

$$X= [(A-B) \times 0.004157 \times T \times 100 \times M_1] / [W \times M_2] \%$$

式中，X为样品中鞣质的含量（%）；A为KMnO$_4$的用量（mL）；B为空白溶液测定中所用的KMnO$_4$的用量（mL）；T为稀释度；W为取样量（g）；M_1为滴定用KMnO$_4$的毫摩尔数；M_2为0.1 mol/L KMnO$_4$的毫摩尔数。

（2）干酪素法

① 标准曲线的制备：精密称取经80℃干燥2小时的鞣酸，配制成0.1mg/mL的30%甲醇溶液。精密吸取1.0mL、2.0mL、3.0mL、4.0mL和5.0mL分别置于10mL棕色量瓶中，用30%甲醇稀释至5mL，加pH 5.0醋酸–醋酸钠缓冲液至刻度，摇匀。

精密吸取上述各溶液1.0mL，分别置于10mL棕色量瓶中，各加Folin试剂0.5mL，混匀，再加5%的碳酸钠溶液至刻度，摇匀。于室温放置20分钟后，以水为空白，在720nm处测定吸光度。以吸光度为纵坐标，浓度为横坐标，绘制标准曲线。

② 样品溶液的制备及测定：称取各炮制品粗粉0.4g，精密称定，置于100mL圆底烧瓶中，加30mL 30%甲醇回流提取1小时，滤过，药渣用20mL 30%甲醇提取2次，每次30分钟，滤过，合并3次滤液，并将其置于100mL量瓶中，药渣用30%甲醇洗涤3次，每次5mL，合并洗液和滤液，用30%甲醇稀释至刻度，摇匀。

精密吸取上述溶液3mL，置于25mL量瓶中，加pH 5.0的醋酸–醋酸钠缓冲液10mL、30%甲醇7mL，混匀，得溶液Ⅰ。

精密吸取溶液Ⅰ 10mL，置于已盛有250mg干酪素的50mL棕色量瓶中，在震荡器上震荡1小时，滤过，滤液摇匀，即得溶液Ⅱ。

分别吸取溶液Ⅰ和Ⅱ各1.0mL，置于10mL棕色量瓶中，依"标准曲线的制备"项下的方法，自"各加Folin试剂0.5mL"起依法测定吸光度，测得吸光度A_1和A_2，依两吸光度之差（ΔA），求出鞣质的量，计算出样品中的含量。

$$X（\%）= (100 \times CT) / (W \times 10^6) \%$$

式中，C为样品溶液的浓度（μg/mL）；T为稀释度；W为样品重量（g）。

实验指导 •••

1. 预习

（1）测定溶液中为什么要加入硫酸（高锰酸钾法）？

（2）制炭前后芦丁和鞣质的含量有何变化，为什么？

2. 基本操作和操作注意点

（1）炒时铁锅的温度不能超过250℃，槐米温度不能超过210℃。

（2）药材称重时要先拣净杂质；炒后要计算出炭率，出炭率不能低于82%。

（3）药材在研钵中研成粗粉时，生品与制品的粗细要一致。

（4）槐米应该在60℃干燥，芦丁也要在60℃干燥至恒重。

（5）若消耗的高锰酸钾溶液的体积太小，可加倍取样量进行测定。

（6）配制溶液Ⅰ时，样品液、pH 5.0的缓冲液以及30%的甲醇都要精密吸取。

3. 实验报告格式

（1）实验目的

（2）实验原理

（3）实验内容及计算结果

①芦丁的含量测定

表3-1 芦丁的含量测定

样品	$W(g)$	$C(\mu g/mL)$	$X(\%)$
生品			
槐米炭			

②鞣质的含量测定

表3-2 高锰酸钾法

样品	$W(g)$	$A(mL)$	$B(mL)$	$A-B(mL)$	$C(\mu g/mL)$	$X(\%)$
生品						
槐米炭						

表3-3 干酪素法

样品	$W(g)$	A_1	A_2	ΔA	$C(\mu g/mL)$	$X(\%)$
生品						
槐米炭						

（4）讨论

4. 实验后思考

（1）槐米中有哪些成分可以止血？制炭后又有哪些成分可以止血？

（2）槐米的炮制方法还有哪些？制炭有何意义？

（3）炒时温度越高，鞣质含量越多，止血作用增强。是否可因此认为制炭时温度越高越好，为什么？

（4）鞣质的含量测定方法有几种？这些方法有何优缺点？请你设计一种测定槐米中鞣质的方法。

（李 凯 薛鹏飞）

Experiment 3   The Assay of Rutin and Tannin in the Crude and the Processed Sophorae Flos

◆ Experimental purposes

1. To master the assay of Rutin and Tannin.

2. To understand the effects of processing on Sophorae Flos via comparing the contents of rutin and tannin before and after processing.

◆ Experimental principle

Sophorae Flos is the dried flower bud of *Sophora japonica* L. (Fam. Leguminosae) . It can arrest the bleeding by reducing the heat in blood. It is often used in the treatment of hematochezia, hemorrhoidal bleeding, dysentery with bloody stools, abnormal uterine bleeding, spitting of blood and epistaxis. It contains rutin and triterpenic saponin which can be hydrolyzed to betulin, sophoradiol, glucose and glucose half aldehyde. It also includes tannin which has the effects of astringing, inducing astringency, arresting bleeding, dysentery and antisepsis.

According to the system of TCM, it is considered that carbonizing can alleviate the nature of Sophorae Flos, produce the astringency and then strengthen the effect of arresting bleeding. The modern chemical and pharmacological studies have confirmed that the content of tannin could be increased after carbonizing.

This experiment employs the methods of HPLC, potassium permanganate and casein to determine the contents of rutin and tannin.

◆ Experimental apparatus

1. Instruments

HPLC, C_{18} chromatographic column, 100mL conical flask with cover, ultrasonic cleaners, spectrophotometer, pot, iron shovel, enamel plate, water bath, analytical balance, volumetric flask (10mL, 25mL, 100mL, 500mL), 10mL and 50mL amber volumetric flask, measuring cylinder (10mL, 500mL), 100mL round bottom beaker, 10mL suction pipet, acid buret (10mL, 25mL), filter paper, glass rod, separating funnel, beaker, electric furnace, oscillating instrument, Soxhlet's extractor, incipient fusion glass funnel, thermometer (300℃) .

2. Medicinal materials and chemicals

Sophorae Flos, rutin (CRS), tannic acid (CRS), $KMnO_4$, concentrated sulfuric acid, indicarmine, NaCl, $BaSO_4$, gelatin, acetic acid, sodium acetate, cheese, sodium carbonate, tannic acid, sodium tungstate, phosphoric acid, glacial acetic acid (CR) and methanol (CR, AR) .

◆ Experimental content

1. Assay of the content of rutin

1.1 Chromatographic condition: Octadecylsilane bonded silica as a filler, methanol and 1% acetic acid solution (32∶68) as the mobile phase, detection wavelength is 257nm.

1.2 Preparation of reference solution: Weigh the proper amount of rutin, accurately, then add methanol to make the reference solution（containing 0.1mg of rutin per 1mL）.

1.3 Preparation of the test solution：Weigh accurately 0.1g coarse powder of Sophorae Flos and carbonized Sophorae Flos，respectively，to a conical flask with cover，and then add 50mL methanol，ultrasonic extract（power 250W，frequency 25kHz）for 30 minutes. Set aside to cool，complement the loss weight by methanol，mix well and filter. Precisely pipet 2mL filtrate to 10mL volumetric flask，then add methanol to the scale and mix well.

1.4 Determination：precisely inject reference solution and the test solution 10μL respectively into the liquid chromatograph.

2. Assay of the content of tannin

2.1 Method of potassium permanganate

2.1.1 Weigh accurately about 10g coarse powder of Sophorae Flos and carbonized Sophorae Flos，respectively. Add 300mL of distilled water to boil for 30 minutes with general heat and filter. Add 100mL distilled water to extract them twice. Combine the filtrates into a 500mL volumetric flask and dilute with distilled water to scale. Filter and discard the residue after 12h. Pipet accurately 10mL of the filtrate into a 1000mL triangle beaker，add 500mL distilled water，5mL of 0.6% indicarmine and 20mL of sulfuric acid，and then titrate with 0.02 mol/L potassium permanganate solution until yellowish-green appears. Record the volume of the potassium permanganate solution as "A".

2.1.2 Assaying the vacancy solution：Pipet accurately 100mL of the solution above-mentioned, add 30mL gelatin solution prepared justly，saturated with sodium chloride and add 10mL of 10% diluted sulfuric acid and 10g of barium sulfate. After shaking for several minutes，filter with the filter paper. Pipet 10mL of the filtrate and titrate with 0.02mol/L potassium permanganate solution until yellowish-green appears. Record the volume of the potassium permanganate solution as "B".

2.1.3 Calculation of the content of tannin in Flos Sophorae：Take tannic acid as the standard substance and 1mL of 0.1mol/L the potassium permanganate solution corresponds to 0.004157g tannic acid.

$$X = [(A-B) \times 0.004157 \times T \times 100 \times M_1] / [W \times M_2] \%$$

Note：

X：the percentage of tannin（%）；A：the volume of potassium permanganate solution（mL）；B：the volume of potassium permanganate solution in assaying the vacancy solution（mL）；T：the dilution ratio；W：the weight of the sample（g）；M_1：the mmol of the volume of potassium permanganate solution when diluting；M_2：the mmol of the volume of 0.1 mol/L potassium permanganate solution.

2.2 The method of casein

2.2.1 Preparation of reference solution：Measure accurately tannic acid（CRS），previously dried in vacuum to constant weight at 80℃ for 2 hours，to prepare the 30% methanol solution containing 0.1mg tannic acid per 1mL. Transfer accurately 1.0，2.0，3.0，4.0 and 5.0mL，respectively，into a 10mL amber volumetric flask. Dilute with 30% methanol to 5.0mL，and then add pH5.0 acetic acid-sodium acetate buffer to scale and mix well.

Pipet accurately 10mL of the solutions above-mentioned into 10mL amber volumetric flask. Add respectively 0.5mL of Folin regent. After mixing well，add 5% sodium carbonate solution to scale and then mix well. Allow to stand for 20 minutes and measure the absorbance at 720nm，taking distilled water as vacancy. Take the absorbance as ordinate and the concentration as abscissa and plot the standard curve.

2.2.2 Preparation of test solution and assay：Weigh accurately 0.4g coarse powder of Sophorae Flos and carbonized Sophorae Flos，respectively，into 100mL round bottom flask. Add 30mL methanol to extract for 1 hour. Extract the residue with 20mL methanol for 2 times, 30 minutes per time. Filter into a 100mL volumetric flask and wash the residue with 5mL of 30% methanol for 3 times. Combine the washings into the flask and add 30% methanol to scale, and then mix well.

Pipet accurately 3mL of the solutions above-mentioned into a 25mL volumetric flask, add 10mL of pH 5.0 acetic acid-sodium acetate buffer and 7mL of 30% methanol to scale. Mix well and record it as solution Ⅰ.

Pipet accurately 10mL of solution into a 50mL amber volumetric flask containing 250mg casein and shake in the oscillating instrument for 1 hour. Filter and mix well and record it as solution Ⅱ.

Pipet accurately 10mL of solution Ⅰ and Ⅱ into a 10mL amber volumetric flask. Proceed as described under Preparation of standard curve, beginning at the words "add 0.5mL of Folin regent···". Measure the absorbance A_1 and A_2 and calculate the content of tannin on the base of the difference between A_1 and A_2.

$$X(\%) = (100 \times CT)/(W \times 10^6)\%$$

Note:

X: the content of tannin (%); C: the concentration of the test solution (μg/mL); T: the dilution ratio; W: the weight of sample (g).

◆ Experimental instruction

1. Preview

1.1 Why add sulfuric acid into the solution when using the method of potassium permanganate?

1.2 What are the changes in rutin and tannin content before and after carbonizing? Why?

2. Primary operation and the notes of the operation

2.1 The temperature of the iron pan should not be more than 250℃ and the temperature of the Flos Sophorae should be lower than 210℃.

2.2 Remove the foreign matters completely before weighing. Calculate the rate of carbonization and the rate should not be less than 82%.

2.3 The size of the powder of Flos Sophorae and its carbonized degree should be consistent.

2.4 Flos Sophorae should be dried at temperature of 60 ℃ and rutin should be dried to constant weight at 60℃.

2.5 Double the sample when the titrating volume of potassium permanganate solution is less.

2.6 The volume of the test solution, pH 5.0 buffer and 30% methanol solution should be accurate when preparation the solution Ⅰ.

3. Format of the experiment report

3.1 Purpose

3.2 Principle

3.3 Content of the experiment and calculating results

3.3.1 Assaying of the content of rutin

Table 3-1　Assaying of the content of rutin

Sample	$W(g)$	$C(\mu g/mL)$	$X(\%)$
Crude drug			
Processed drug			

3.3.2 The assaying of the content of tannin

Table 3-2　Method of potassium permanganate

Sample	$W(g)$	$A(mL)$	$B(mL)$	$A-B(mL)$	$C(\mu g/mL)$	$X(\%)$
Crude drug						
Processed drug						

Table 3-3　Method of cheese

Sample	$W(g)$	A_1	A_2	ΔA	$C(\mu g/mL)$	$X(\%)$
Crude drug						
Processed drug						

3.4 Discussion

4. Considerations after the experiment

4.1 What constituents can arrest the bleeding? What constitutes can arrest the bleeding after carbonizing?

4.2 What are the other methods of processing? What is the significance of carbonizing?

4.3 The higher temperature, the higher content of tannin and the better effect of arresting the bleeding. So can we think that the higher temperature leads to the better effect when processing, why?

4.4 How many methods to assay the rutin and tannin? What merits and defaults do they have? Please design a method to determine the content of tannin in Flos Sophorae.

（Edited by Kai Li and Pengfei Xue）

实验四　山楂及其炮制品中总有机酸和总黄酮的含量测定

实验目的 •••

1. 掌握山楂中总有机酸和总黄酮含量测定方法。
2. 通过山楂不同炮制品中总有机酸和总黄酮的含量比较，了解山楂炮制的作用和意义。

实验原理 •••

山楂为蔷薇科植物山里红 *Crataegus pinnatifida* Bge. var. *major* N. E. Br. 或山楂 *Crataegus pinnatifida* Bge. 的干燥成熟果实，具消食健胃、行气散瘀、化浊降脂的功效。常用的炮制方法有炒黄、炒焦和炒炭等。山楂经不同方法炮制后，其作用有所改变，如焦山楂善于消食止泻，山楂炭长于止血止泻。现代研究认为，山楂中含有的有机酸和黄酮类化合物具有多方面的药理作用。其中有机酸类能增加胃中消化酶的分泌，促进消化；黄酮类化合物对心血管疾病有显著疗效，可扩张血管、强心、降压和降脂等。

山楂酸，甘、微温，具有酸之偏性。因此，山楂炮制的目的是降低酸性，缓和或减少刺激性。本实验通过山楂炮制前后总有机酸和总黄酮含量的比较，说明山楂的炮制意义。

实验器材 •••

1. 仪器　称量瓶，万分之一分析天平，十万分之一分析天平，锥形瓶，量筒，圆底烧瓶，水浴锅，冷凝管，玻璃漏斗，移液管，容量瓶，吸量管，碱式滴定管，磁力搅拌器，电磁炉，紫外分光光度计。

2. 药材及试剂　山楂，焦山楂，氢氧化钠，酚酞，滤纸，乙醇，亚硝酸钠，硝酸铝，芦丁对照品。

实验内容 •••

1. 总有机酸含量测定　称取样品细粉各约1g，精密称定，分别精密加入水100mL，室温下浸泡4小时，时时振摇，滤过。精密量取续滤液25mL，加水50mL，加酚酞指示液2滴，用0.1 mol/L的氢氧化钠滴定，即得。每1mL 0.1mol/L氢氧化钠滴定液相当于6.404mg的枸橼酸（总有机酸含量以枸橼酸计）。

2. 总黄酮含量测定

（1）对照品溶液的制备　精密称取芦丁对照品25mg，置50mL量瓶中，加乙醇适量，超声处理使溶解，放冷，加乙醇至刻度，摇匀。精密量取20mL，置50mL量瓶中，加水至刻度，摇匀，即得（0.2mg/mL）。

（2）标准曲线的制备　精密量取对照品溶液0mL、1mL、2mL、3mL、4mL、5mL，分别置10mL量瓶中，各加30%乙醇至5mL，加5%亚硝酸钠溶液0.3mL，摇匀，放置6分钟，加10%硝酸铝溶液0.3mL，摇匀，放置6分钟，加氢氧化钠试液4mL，再加水至刻度，振摇，放置15分钟，以相应试剂为空白，立即照紫外–可见分光光度计法，在500nm的波长处测定吸光度（A），以吸光度（A）为纵坐标，浓度C（mg/mL）为横坐标。

（3）测定方法　称取山楂生品和炮制品细粉各约1g，精密称定，分别置圆底烧瓶中，加乙醇

20mL，置水浴上回流 1.5 小时，放冷后，滤过，精密吸取续滤液 2mL，置 10mL 量瓶中，加 60% 乙醇至刻度，摇匀，照标准曲线制备项下的方法，自"加 30% 乙醇至 5mL"起依法测定吸光度，根据标准曲线计算供试品溶液中芦丁的浓度，并换算成样品中总黄酮的含量。

实验指导 ●●●

1. 基本操作和操作注意点

（1）基本操作　掌握总有机酸和总黄酮的测定方法。

（2）操作注意点　① 山楂应去尽核。② 酸碱滴定时要注意滴定管检漏。③ 紫外分光光度计应事先预热。

2. 实验报告格式

（1）实验目的

（2）实验原理

（3）实验数据及计算结果

表 4-1　总有机酸含量

样品	重量（g）	消耗 NaOH 毫升数	百分含量（%）
生品			
炮制品			

表 4-2　总黄酮含量

样品	重量（g）	吸光度（A）	百分含量（%）
生品			
炮制品			

（4）讨论

3. 实验后思考

（1）山楂主要含哪些有机酸类及黄酮类化合物？

（2）有机酸类和黄酮类化合物的含量测定方法还有哪些？

（3）山楂的不同炮制方法是否有意义？

（张春凤　孙小雅　薛鹏飞）

Experiment 4　The Assay of Total Organic Acid and Total Flavones in the Crude and the Processed Crataegi Fructus

◆ Experimental purposes

1. To master the assay of total organic acid and total flavonoes.

2. To study the action and the processing significance of Crataegi Fructus by comparing the content of total organic acid and total flavonoes before and after processing.

◆ Experimental principle

Crataegi Fructus is the dried ripe fruit of *Crataegus pinnatifida* Bge. var *major* N. E. Br., or *Crataegus pinnatifida* Bge. The drug is collected in autumn when the fruit is ripe, cut into slices, and dried. The drug has the functions of stimulating digestion and promoting the functional activity of the stomach, improving the normal flow of *qi* and dissipating blood stasis, lowering lipid. The usual processing methods of Crataegi Fructus include stir-frying Crataegi Frucms, charring Crataegi Fructus and charcoaling Crataegi Fructus. The traditional Chinese medicine thinks that its functions will change after different methods of processing, for example, charred Crataegi Frucms shines in digestion and its charcoal shines in convergence and hemostasis.

Modern research shows that the flavones and organic acids of Crataegi Fructus possess multifarious pharmacological actions. Of which, the organic acid can strengthen the digestive-enzymic secernent of stomach, and promote digestion. Crataegi Fructus can also intensify the activities of the gastric lipase and peptidase. The flavones are effective in the treatment of cardiovascular disease, via expanding blood vessel, decreasing blood pressure and fat, and its cardiotonic activity.

Taste sweet, slight warmth, and sourness are the properties of crataegolic acid. Therefore, the purposes of the processing of Crataegi Frucms are decreasing sourness, alleviating or reducing its irritation. The experiment will show that the processing of Crataegi Fructus has great significance through comparing the contents of the flavones and organic acids after and before processing.

◆ Experimental apparatus

1. Instruments

Weighing bottle, 1/10000 analytic balance, 1/100000 analytic balance, conical beaker, dosimeter, round bottom flask, water-bath cauldron, condensation tube, hyalo-funnel, transferring pipette, volumetric flask, pipette, basic burette, magnetic stirrer, induction cooker, UV spectrophotometer.

2. Medicinal materials and chemicals

Crataegi Fructus, sodium hydroxide, phenolphthalein, filter paper, alcohol (AR), sodium nitrite, aluminium nitrate, rutin (SR).

◆ Experimental content

1. Assay of the total organic acid

Weigh 1g of the fine powder, accurately. Add 100mL of water, then soak for 4 hours at room temperature, shaking constantly and filter. Pipet 25mL of the filtrate accurately, 50mL of water and 2 drops of phenolphthalein.

The organic acid is titrated with sodium hydroxide（0.1mol/L）VS，and then calculate the content. Each mL of sodium hydroxide（0.1mol/L）VS is equivalent to 6.404mg of citric acid（$C_6H_8O_7$）. The content of total organic acids is calculated as citric acid（$C_6H_8O_7$）.

2. Assay of the total flavones

2.1 Preparation of standard curve

Accurately weight 25mg of Rutin to a 50mL of the volumetric flask，add proper amount of ethanol，and ultrasonic to dissolve，let cool，add ethanol to the scale，mix well. Pipet 20mL of the solution accurately to a 50mL of volumetric flask，dilute it to scale with distilled water，shake up and reserve（0.2mg/1mL）.

2.2 Preparation of standard curve

Pipet 0，1.0，2.0，3.0，4.0，5.0mL of the above-mentioned standard solution accurately to 10mL volumetric flask and add 30% of ethanol to 5.0mL，add 0.3mL of 5% sodium nitrate solution accurately，and shake up. 6 minutes later，add 0.3mL of 10% aluminium nitrate again，shake up，after 6 minutes，add 4mL of sodium hydroxide test solution and dilute to the graduation with distilled water，mix well，stand for 15 minutes. Determine the absorbance（A）at 500nm，using A as the ordinate，standard solution concentration（C）as the abscissa to get the standard curve.

2.3 Assay of sample

Accurately weigh 1g fine powder of the crude and processed sample to the round bottom flasks，add 20mL of ethyl alcohol，reflux 1.5 hours in water-bath，filter after cooling. Accurately transfer 2mL of the filtrate to a 10mL of volumetric flask，add 60% ethyl alcohol to the scale，and mix well. Determine the absorbance of samples as the method described above，and calculate the content of the total flavones.

◆ Experimental instruction

1. Primary operation and the notes of the operation

1.1 Primary operation

Master the determining methods of the total flavones and organic acids.

1.2 Operating notes

1.2.1 The foreign matters and fallen kernels of Crataegi Fructus should be removed.

1.2.2 Pay attention to leak detection in acid-base titration.

1.2.3 UV spectrophotometer should be preheated.

2. Format of the experiment report

2.1 Purpose

2.2 Principle

2.3 Experimental data and calculating results

2.3.1 Assay of the total organic acid

Table 4-1　Assay of the total organic acid

Sample	Weight（g）	Consumable NaOH（mL）	Content（%）
Crude drug			
Processed drug			

2.3.2 Assay of the total flavones

Table 4-2 Assay of the total flavones

Sample	Weight (g)	Absorbance (A)	Content (%)
Crude drug			
Processed drug			

2.4 Discussion

3. Considerations after the experiment

3.1 Which kind of compounds do the organic acids and flavones belong to?

3.2 What other methods can we use to determine their contents?

3.3 Whether is the different processing of Crataegi Fructus meaningful?

（Edited by Chunfeng Zhang，Xiaoya Sun and Pengfei Xue）

实验五 骨碎补及其炮制品中黄酮的含量测定

实验目的 ●••

1. 掌握采用分光光度法测定骨碎补不同炮制品中总黄酮含量的方法和高效液相色谱法测定骨碎补不同炮制品中柚皮苷含量的方法。

2. 通过比较骨碎补炮制前后柚皮苷和总黄酮类成分的含量，了解炮制对骨碎补的作用和意义。

实验原理 ●••

骨碎补为水龙骨科植物槲蕨 *Drynaria fortunei*（Kunze）J. Sm. 的干燥根茎，具补肾强骨，续伤止痛之功效。用于肾虚腰痛，耳鸣耳聋，牙齿松动，跌扑损伤等症。骨碎补质地坚硬，砂烫后质地酥脆，有效成分易被溶出。现代研究认为，砂烫骨碎补与生骨碎补相比，能明显提高其活性成分柚皮苷等二氢黄酮类化合物的溶出率。

骨碎补中的二氢黄酮类化合物紫外光谱的最大吸收位于281nm左右，与柚皮苷的最大吸收283nm基本一致，因此，可用紫外分光光度法，以柚皮苷为对照品，283nm为测定波长，测定总黄酮含量，以此为指标考察砂烫对骨碎补有效成分的影响，说明骨碎补的炮制意义。

实验器材 ●••

1. **仪器** 索氏提取器，100mL圆底烧瓶2只，100mL容量瓶2只，50mL容量瓶1只，25mL容量瓶2只，10mL容量瓶6只，水浴锅，紫外分光光度计，分析天平，粉碎机。

2. **药材及试剂** 骨碎补，砂烫骨碎补，柚皮苷对照品，甲醇，称量纸，滤纸，脱脂棉。

实验内容 ●••

1. **总黄酮含量测定**

（1）标准曲线的制备 精密称取柚皮苷对照品5mg，置50mL容量瓶中，甲醇定容至刻度，作为对照品溶液备用。精密吸取上述对照品溶液0.5mL、1.0mL、1.5mL、2.0mL、2.5mL、3.0mL于10mL容量瓶中，用甲醇定容至刻度，以甲醇为空白，在283nm处测吸收度（A），并以吸收度A为纵坐标，对照品溶液浓度C（mg/mL）为横坐标，经回归得标准曲线方程。

（2）样品溶液制备及测定 精密称取骨碎补炮制品与生品粉末各1g，分别置索氏提取器中，用50mL甲醇提取2小时，将提取液转移至100mL容量瓶中，以甲醇定容至刻度，精密吸取2mL置于25mL容量瓶中，以甲醇定容至刻度，作为待测液。于283nm处测定吸收度，按回归方程计算待测液中总黄酮浓度C（mg/mL），并换算成总黄酮百分含量。

2. **柚皮苷含量的测定**

（1）色谱条件 以十八烷基硅烷键合硅胶为填充剂；以甲醇–醋酸–水（35∶4∶65）为流动相；检测波长为283nm。理论板数按柚皮苷峰计算应不低于3000。

（2）对照品溶液的制备 取柚皮苷对照品适量，精密称定，加甲醇制成每1mL含柚皮苷60μg的溶液，即得。

（3）供试品溶液的制备 分别取骨碎补生品和炮制品粗粉各0.25g，精密称定，置锥形瓶中，加甲醇30mL，加热回流3小时，放冷，滤过，滤液置50mL量瓶中，用少量甲醇分数次洗涤容器，洗液滤入同一量瓶中，加甲醇至刻度摇匀，即得。

（4）测定法 分别精密吸取对照品溶液与供试品溶液各10μL注入液相色谱仪，测定，计算待测液中柚皮苷浓度，并计算生制品柚皮苷的百分含量。

实验指导 ●●●

1.基本操作和注意事项

（1）基本操作 掌握骨碎补中总黄酮含量的测定方法。

（2）注意事项 ①骨碎补应去净茸毛；②分光光度计应事先预热稳定。

2.实验报告格式

（1）实验目的

（2）实验原理

（3）实验内容及计算结果

①骨碎补的炮制

②总黄酮的含量测定

表5-1 总黄酮的含量测定

样品	样品重量（g）	吸收度（A）	浓度（μg/mL）	百分含量（%）
生品骨碎补				
砂烫骨碎补				

③柚皮苷的含量测定

表5-2 柚皮苷的含量测定

样品	样品重量（g）	峰面积	浓度（μg/mL）	百分含量（%）
生品骨碎补				
砂烫骨碎补				

（4）讨论

3.实验后思考

（1）骨碎补主要含哪些黄酮类化合物？

（2）黄酮类化合物的含量测定方法还有哪些？

（张春凤 孙小雅 薛鹏飞）

Experiment 5 The Assay of Flavones in the Crude and the Processed Drynariae Rhizoma

◆ Experimontal Purposes

1. To master the assaying method of total flavones and naringin in Drynariae Rhizoma by UV-spectmphotometry and HPLC.

2. To learn the functions and meanings of processing by comparing the contents change of the total flavones and naringin in Drynaxiae Rhizoma and Drynariae Rhizoma（sand scalding）.

◆ Experimental principle

Drynariae Rhizoma is the dried rhizome of *Drynaria fortunei*（Kunze）J. Sm. With the actions of replenishing the kidney, strengthening the bones, promoting the healing of fracture, and relieving pain, it is used to treat deficiency syndrome of the kidney marked by back pain, tinnitus, impairment of hearing and looseness of teeth, tramatic injury, bone fracture, external use for alopecia areata and vitiligo. After been scalded, Drynariae Rhizoma becomes loose and friable, and more of the effective components can be dissolved.

The flavones in Drynariae Rhizoma have the most strong absorption at about 281nm, according with naringin, so we carry out UV-spectmphotometry, using naringin as CRS, 283nm as absorption wavelength, to measure the content of the total flavones. Moreover, the action of scalding to Drynariae Rhizoma can be explained by comparing the change contents of the total flavones in different Drynariae Rhizoma.

◆ Experimental apparatus

1. Instruments

Soxhlet's extractor, round bottom flask（100mL × 2）, volumetric flask（100mL × 2; 50mL × 1; 25mL × 2; 10mL × 6）, analytical balance, water bath, UV-spectrophotometer, pulverizer, weight paper, filter paper, cotton.

2. Medicinal materials and chemicals

Drynariae Rhizoma, sand, methanol（AR）, redistilled water, naringin CRS.

◆ Experimental content

1. Assay of total flavones

1.1 Preparation of reference curve: Accurately weigh 5mg naringin CRS to a 50mL volumetric flask, add methanol to the scale as reference solutions. Pipet accurately the reference solution 0.5, 1.0, 1.5, 2.0, 2.5, 3.0mL to six 10mL volumetric flasks, add methanol to scale. Use methanol as blank, and measure the absorbance at 283 nm. Take the absorbance as Y-coordinate and the concentrations of the reference solutions as abscissa, and get the regression equation.

1.2 Preparation and determination of the solution of test sample: Accurately weigh 1 g powder［Drynariae Rhizoma（scalding）and Drynariae Rhizoma］to 2 Soxhlet's extractors, extract for 2 hours with 50mL methanol, transfer the extractors to 100mL volumetric flasks, add methanol to scale. Pipet accurately 2mL to 25mL volumetric flasks, add methanol to scale as test solution. Measure the absorbance at 283nm, calculate the contents（ C ： mg/mL ）and convert it to the content of the total flavones.

2. Assay of naringin

2.1 Chromatographic system and system suitability：Use octadecylsilane bonded silica gel as the stationary phase and methanol-acetic acid-water（35：4：65）as the mobile phase. The detector is set at 283nm. The number of theoretical plates of the column is not less than 3000, calculated with the reference to the peak of naringin.

2.2 Preparation of reference solution：Weigh accurately 3mg naringin CRS in a 50mL volumetric flask. Dissolve and dilute with methanol to scale and mix well.

2.3 Preparation of test solution：Weigh nearly 3g the crude and processed Drynariae Rhizoma, make into coarse powder and accurately weigh 0.25g of power respectively in a conical flask. Add 30mL methanol and heat under reflux for 3 hours. Transfer the solution into a 50mL volumetric flask, wash the vessels with some methanol and transfer the washings to the volumetric flask. Dilute with methanol to scale and mix well.

2.4 Procedures：Accurately inject 10μL the reference solution and the test solution, respectively, into the column, determinate and calculate the content.

◆ Experimental instruction

1. Primary operations and notes of the operations

1.1 Primary operations

Grasp the method of assaying the total flavones in Drynariae Rhizoma.

1.2 Notes of operations

1.2.1 Remove root hatrs entirely.

1.2.2 Warm-up the UV-spectrophotometer before measuring.

2. Format of the experiment report

2.1 Purpose

2.2 Principle

2.3 Contents and results

2.3.1 Processing

2.3.2 Assay

Table 5-1　Content of total flavonoids

Sample	Weight（g）	Absorbance（A）	Concentration（μg/mL）	Content（%）
Drynariae Rhizoma				
Drynariae Rhizoma（scalding）				

Table 5-2　Content of naringin

Sample	Weight（g）	Peak area	Concentration（μg/mL）	Content（%）
Drynariae Rhizoma				
Drynariae Rhizoma（scalding）				

2.4 Discussion

3. Considerations after the experiment

3.1 What are the flavones in Drynariae Rhizoma?

3.2 What are the other methods of assaying flavone?

（Edited by Chunfeng Zhang，Xiaoya Sun and Pengfei Xue）

实验六 枳壳及其炮制品中总挥发油的含量测定

实验目的 ●●●

1. 掌握挥发油含量测定方法。

2. 了解麸炒对枳壳挥发油含量的影响及其炮制作用。

实验原理 ●●●

枳壳为芸香科植物酸橙 *Citrus aurantium* L. 及其栽培变种的干燥未成熟果实。性微寒，味苦、辛、酸。归脾、胃经。具理气宽中，行滞消胀之效。用于胸胁气滞，胀满疼痛，食积不化，痰饮内停，脏器下垂等。

生枳壳作用较强，可行气宽中除胀，麸炒后减低其刺激性，缓和燥性和酸性，增强健脾消胀作用。因其作用缓和，宜用于年老体弱而气滞者。本实验采用挥发油测定器，对炮制前后枳壳中总挥发油的含量进行测定，进而说明炮制的意义。

实验器材 ●●●

1 仪器 分析天平，烧杯，圆底烧瓶，挥发油测定器，量筒，比重计，电热套等。

2 药材及辅料 枳壳，麸炒枳壳等。

实验内容 ●●●

1. 总挥发油含量测定 精密称取枳壳生品及炮制品粉末（过2~3号筛）各50g（精确至0.01g），分别置1000mL圆底烧瓶中，加水300~500mL（或适量）与玻璃珠数粒，振摇混合后，连接挥发油测定器与冷凝管。自冷凝管上端加水直至使其充满挥发油测定器的刻度部分，并溢流入烧瓶为止。置电热套上缓缓加热至沸，并保持微沸约5小时，至测定器中油量不再增加，停止加热，放置片刻，开启测定器下端的活塞，将水缓缓放出，至油层上端到达刻度零线上面5mm处为止。放置1小时以上，再开启活塞使油层下降至其上端恰与刻度零线平齐，读取挥发油量，并计算供试品中挥发油中的含量（%）。

2. 挥发油比重的测定 取洁净干燥至恒重的比重管，精密吸取1mL挥发油加入比重管中，在25℃水浴中保持10分钟，使油面至刻度，取出擦干，精密称重，反复3次，取平均值为挥发油重，以同样方法求出水重，并按下式计算。

$$比重 = (W_2 - W_0) \rho / (W_1 - W_0)$$

式中，W_0 为比重管重；W_1 为比重管加水重；W_2 为比重管加油重；ρ 为25℃时水的比重。

实验指导 ●●●

1. 基本操作和操作注意点

（1）基本操作 ①掌握挥发油含量测定方法。②掌握挥发油比重的测定方法。

（2）操作注意点 ①挥发油测定装置的各连接部位应密封，以免挥发油损失。②在读取挥发油量时，应静置一段时间，使其充分与水分层。③比重管须恒重。④挥发油在测定其物理常数前，应脱水处理。

2. 实验报告格式

（1）实验目的

（2）实验原理

（3）实验数据及计算结果

表6-1　挥发油的含量

样品	挥发油含量（%）	比重（d）
生品		
炮制品		

（4）讨论

3. 实验后思考

（1）根据你所查阅的文献，谈谈枳壳炮制前后药理作用有何变化？

（2）通过对枳壳生品和炮制品中总挥发油的定量测定实验，说明了什么？

（李　飞　颜家壬　薛鹏飞）

Experiment 6 The Assay of Volatile Oil in the Crude and the Processed Aurantii Fructus

◆ Experimental purposes

1. To master the assay of volatile oil in Aurantii Fructus.

2. To investigate the effect of bran stir-frying on the content of volatile oil in Aurantii Fructus and its processing effect.

◆ Experimental principle

Aurantii Fructus is the immature dried fruit of *Citrus aurantium* L. and its cultivated varieties (Fam. Rutaceae). It is slightly cold in nature, bitter, acrid and sour in taste, distributes to spleen and stomach channel. The functions of Aurantii Fructus are regulating the flow of qi, removing the stagnation, and alleviating distension. The indications are distension and pain in the chest and hypochondriac regions due to stagnation of qi, indigestion with retention of phlegm and fluid, splanchnoptosis, etc.

The function of crude drug is stronger than processed drug. It can be used to eliminate stagnation of qi and relieve stuffiness sensation in the chest and abdomen. After stir-frying with bran, the stimulation of the drug will be lower, its dryness nature and acidity will be mild, and its function of invigorating the spleen and relieve stuffiness sensation in chest and abdomen will be enhanced. Therefore, the processed drug is suitable for the old patients who suffer stagnation of qi.

This experiment adopts volatile oil determination apparatus to determinate its content in the crude drug and processed drug, then to explain the significance of processing.

◆ Experimental apparatus

1. Instruments

Analytical balance, beaker, round bottom flask, volatile oil determination apparatus, measuring cylinder, electric heating sleeve, gravimeter, etc.

2. Medicinal materials and chemicals

Aurantii Fructus, Processed Aurantii Fructus, etc.

◆ Experimental content

1. Determination of volatile oil

Weigh exactly 50g powder (to the nearest 0.01g) of crude drug and processed drug (pass through No.2 or No.3 sieves and then mix well) and put them into 1000mL round bottom flasks respectively. Add 300-500mL water and a few glass beads, shake and mix well. Connect flask to volatile oil determination tube and condensing tube. Add water through the top of condensing tube until the graduated portion is filled and overflows to the flask. Heat the flask gently in an electric heating sleeve or other suitable heating apparatus until boiling and keep boiling for about 5 hours, until the volume of oil does not raise. Stop heating, allow it to stand for a few minutes, and open the stopcock at lower, run off the water layer slowly until the oily layer is 5mm above the zero mark. Stand for at least 1 hour, open the stopcock again, run off the remaining water layer carefully until the oily layer is just on the zero mark. Read the volume of oil in the graduated portion of the tube, and calculate the content of volatile oil, expressed as percentage.

2. Specific gravity test of volatile oil

Pipet exactly 1mL volatile oil in a pycnometer (clean and dry to constant weight). Put the pycnometer in 25℃ water bath, make the oily layer is just on the mark, after 10 minutes, take it out, clean and dry it, measure it accurately, repeat the preceding operation 3 times, and calculate the average weight of volatile oil. Get the weight of water in the same way.

$$\text{Specific gravity} = (W_2 - W_0)\rho / (W_1 - W_0)$$

Note:

W_0: the weight of pycnometer; W_1: the weight of pycnometer and water; W_2: the weight of pycnometer and volatile oil; ρ: the specific gravity of water at 25℃.

◆ Experimental instruction

1. Primary operations and notes of the operations

1.1 Primary operation

1.1.1 Master the determination method the quantity of volatile oil.

1.1.2 Master the determination method the specific gravity of volatile oil.

1.2 Notes of operations

1.2.1 Seal the connect part of the apparatus to avoid the emitting of volatile oil.

1.2.2 Wait for a few minutes to allow the water layer separate thoroughly from the oily layer, and then read the volume of oil in the graduated portion of the tube.

1.2.3 Pycnometer must be constant weight.

1.2.4 Volatile oil should be dehydrated before its physical constant is determinated.

2. Format of the experiment report

2.1 Purpose

2.2 Principle

2.3 Experimental data and calculating results

Table 6-1　Content of volatile oil

Sample	The volume of oil (%)	Specific gravity (d)
Crude drug		
Processed drug		

2.4 Discussion

3. Considerations after the experiment

3.1 Please describe the changes of pharmacological actions after processing, according to the reports that you read.

3.2 What does the assay of volatile oil of crude and processed drug explain?

（Edited by Fei Li, Jiaren Yan and Pengfei Xue）

第三章　炙　法

实验七　炙法代表药物炮制

实验目的 ●●●

1. 掌握酒炙、醋炙、盐炙、姜炙、蜜炙、油炙的操作方法、注意事项及成品质量。
2. 了解酒炙、醋炙、盐炙、姜炙、蜜炙、油炙的目的和意义。

实验原理 ●●●

将净选或切制后的药物加入一定量的液体辅料，用文火拌炒，使辅料逐渐渗入药物组织内部的炮制方法称为炙法。

清代张仲岩在《修事指南》中指出："炙者取中和之性"。药物加液体辅料经加热炒制后，在性味、功效、作用趋势、归经等方面均能发生某些变化，起到增强疗效、降低毒性、抑制偏性、矫臭矫味等作用，从而更好地满足临床用药的需求。

根据所用液体辅料的不同，炙法可以分为酒炙、醋炙、盐炙、蜜炙、姜炙、油炙等法，传统上的炙法以炒炙为主，现代生产中亦有采用烘炙代替炒炙。

1. 酒炙的作用　①改变药性，引药上行；②增强活血通络作用；③矫臭矫味，如乌梢蛇、蕲蛇、紫河车等。

2. 醋炙的作用　①引药入肝，增强疗效；②降低毒性，缓和药性；③矫臭矫味。

3. 盐炙的作用　①引药下行，增强疗效；②增强滋阴降火作用；③缓和药物辛燥之性。

4. 蜜炙的作用　①增强润肺止咳的作用，如百部、冬花、紫菀；②增强补脾益气的作用，如黄芪、甘草、党参等；③缓和药性，如麻黄等。

5. 姜炙的作用　①缓和药物寒性，增强和胃止呕作用；②降低不良反应，增强疗效。

6. 油炙的作用　①增强疗效；②利于粉碎。

实验器材 ●●●

1. 仪器　炒锅，锅铲，电磁炉，搪瓷盘，电子称，烧杯，量杯，玻璃棒等。

2. 药材及试剂　黄酒，米醋，食盐，姜，蜂蜜，食用油，当归，白芍，黄芩，芫花，元胡，杜仲，黄柏，知母，厚朴，竹茹，黄芪，百合，枇杷叶，淫羊藿。

实验内容 ●●●

1. 酒炙法 ⓔ微课1

（1）当归　取净当归饮片，加入定量黄酒拌匀，闷润至酒被吸尽，置热锅内，文火加热，炒至深黄色，取出，晾凉。每100kg当归片，用黄酒10kg。

（2）白芍　取净白芍饮片，加入定量黄酒拌匀，闷润至酒被吸尽，置热锅内，文火加热，炒至微黄色，取出，晾凉。每100kg白芍片，用黄酒10kg。

（3）黄芩　取净黄芩饮片，加入定量黄酒拌匀，闷润至酒被吸尽，置热锅内，文火加热，炒至深黄色，取出，晾凉。每100kg黄芩片，用黄酒10kg。

2. 醋炙法 ⓔ微课2

（1）芫花　取净芫花，加定量米醋拌匀，闷润至醋被吸尽，置热锅内，文火炒至微干，表面灰褐色，放凉。每100kg芫花，用米醋30kg。

（2）延胡索　取净延胡索片，加入定量米醋拌匀，闷润至醋被吸尽，置热锅内，文火加热，炒至深黄色，取出，放凉。每100kg延胡索片，用米醋20kg。

3. 盐炙法 ⓔ微课3

（1）杜仲　取杜仲丝或块，加盐水拌匀，闷透，置热锅内，用文火加热，炒至颜色加深、有焦斑、丝易断时，取出，晾凉。每100 kg杜仲丝或块，用食盐2kg。

（2）黄柏　取黄柏丝或块，加盐水拌匀，闷透，置热锅内，用文火加热，炒至颜色变深、有焦斑时，取出，晾凉。每100kg黄柏丝或块，用食盐2kg。

（3）知母　取净知母片，置热锅内，用文火加热，炒至颜色变深，喷淋盐水，炒干，取出，晾凉。每100kg知母片，用食盐2kg。

4. 姜炙 ⓔ微课4

（1）厚朴　取净厚朴丝，加姜汁拌匀，闷润，待姜汁被吸尽后，置热锅内，用文火炒干，取出，摊晾。每100kg厚朴用生姜10kg。

（2）竹茹　取净竹茹，加姜汁拌匀，闷润，待姜汁被吸尽后，置热锅内，用文火炒至微黄色，取出，摊晾。每100kg竹茹用生姜10kg。

5. 蜜炙 ⓔ微课5

（1）黄芪　取沸水稀释的炼蜜，加入黄芪片拌匀，稍闷，置热锅内，用文火炒至深黄色，不粘手时取出，摊晾。每100kg黄芪用炼蜜25kg。

（2）百合　取净百合，置热锅内，用文火炒至颜色加深时，加沸水稀释过的炼蜜，迅速翻炒均匀，用文火炒至微黄色，不粘手时取出，摊晾。每100kg百合用炼蜜5kg。

（3）枇杷叶　取沸水稀释的炼蜜，加入枇杷叶丝拌匀，闷透，置热锅内，文火炒至微黄色不粘手，取出摊晾。每100kg枇杷叶用炼蜜20kg。

6. 油炙 ⓔ微课6

淫羊藿　先将羊脂油置锅内加热熔化，然后倒入淫羊藿丝，用文火炒至微黄色，取出放凉。每100kg淫羊藿用羊脂油20kg。

实验指导 ●●●

1. 基本操作和操作注意点

（1）采用先拌辅料后炒药的方法时，辅料要与药物拌匀，闷润至被吸尽或渗透到药物组织内部后再炒制。

（2）酒炙药物闷润时，容器要加盖密闭，以防酒迅速挥发。

（3）溶解食盐时，水的用量一般以食盐量的4~5倍为宜。

（4）制备姜汁时，一般以所得姜汁与生姜为1∶1为宜。

（5）蜜炙时间可稍长，尽量除去水分，避免发霉；并注意放凉后密闭贮存。

（6）若液体辅料用量较少，不易与药物拌匀时，可先加适量开水稀释，以利拌匀润制药物。

（7）炙法大多用文火炒制，需勤翻动，使药物受热均匀，炒至规定程度。

（8）先炒制后加辅料的药物，辅料要均匀喷洒在药物上，不要沿锅壁加入，以免辅料迅速蒸发。

（9）炙时，火力不可过大，宜勤翻动，一般炒至近干，颜色加深时，即可出锅摊晾。

2. 实验报告格式

（1）实验目的

（2）实验原理

（3）实验内容

（4）讨论

3. 思考题

（1）各种炙法有何异同点？

（2）知母等药物为何采用先炒药后加辅料的方法炮炙？

（3）蜜炙、姜炙、盐炙、羊油脂炙法所用辅料如何制备？

（4）百合为何采用先炒制后加辅料的方法炮制？

（5）稀释炼蜜时为何需要用沸水？

（季　德　郭常润　赵雅兰）

书网融合……

微课1　　　　微课2　　　　微课3　　　　微课4　　　　微课5　　　　微课6

Experiment 7　Representative Drug Processed by Stir-frying with Liquid Adjuvant

◆ Experimental purposes

1. To master the operation methods, precautions and product quality of stir-frying drug with wine, vinegar, salt, ginger juice, honey and oil.

2. To understand the purpose and significance of stir-frying drug with wine, vinegar, salt, ginger juice, honey and oil.

◆ Experimental principle

The stir-frying drug with liquid adjuvant refers to the method of adding a certain amount of liquid adjuvant to the drug after it has been selected or cut, and stirring it with a civil fire so that the adjuvant gradually penetrates into the internal tissues of the drug.

Zhang Zhongyan of the Qing dynasty pointed out in his *Xiu Shi Zhi Nan*: sizzling to take the nature of neutral. Drug plus liquid adjuvant after heating and frying, in the nature of taste, efficacy, tendency of action, attribution and other aspects can be some changes to enhance the efficacy, reduce toxicity, inhibit bias, odor correction and other effects, so as to better meet the requirements of clinical use of drug.

According to the different liquid adjuvant used, stir-frying drug with liquid adjuvant can be divided into stir-frying drug with wine, vinegar, salt, water diluted honey, ginger, and oil. Traditionally, the sizzling method to stir-frying is primary, while modern production is also used to baking instead of stir-frying.

1. The purpose of stir-frying with wine　A. To change drug effect; B. To enhance blood circulation and dredge meridians; C. To remove the bad odor of some drugs, like Zaocys dhumnades, agkistrodon snake, etc.

2. The role of stir-frying with vinegar　A. To lead the effects of drug to the liver meridian to strengthen the effects; B. To reduce the toxicity of drug and moderate the properties of drug; C. To remove the bad odor of some drugs.

3. The effect of stir-frying with salt　A. To conduct the effects of drug to the kidney meridian and enhance the effects; B. To strengthen the effects of nourishing yin deficiency and purge away fire; C. To moderate the properties of dryness in drug.

4. The function of stir-frying with honey　A. To strengthen the effect of moistening lung to stop cough; B. To enhance the effect of tonifying the spleen and invigorating *qi*; C. To mitigate drug effect.

5. The purpose of stir-frying with ginger juice　A. To alleviate coldness of drug, and soothe the stomach to arrest vomit; B. To reduce side effects and enhance its efficacy.

6. The purpose of stir-frying with oil　A. To enhance efficacy; B. To facilitate crushing.

◆ Experimental apparatus

1. Instruments

Wok, spatula, electric stove, enameled tray, electronic scale, beaker, measuring glass and glass rod, etc.

2. Medicinal materials and chemicals

Wine, rice vinegar, salt, ginger, honey, cooking oil; Angelicae Sinensis Radix, Paeoniae Radix Alba, Scutellariae Radix, Genkwa Flos, Corydalis Rhizoma, Eucommiae Cortex, Phellodendri Chinensis Cortex, Anemarrhenae Rhizoma, Magnoliae Officinalis Cortex, Bambusae Caulis in Taenias, Astragali Radix, Lilii Bulbus, Eriobotryae Folium, Epimedii Folium.

◆ Experimental content

1. Stir-frying with wine

1.1 Angelicae Sinensis Radix (Danggui)

Mix the clean slices of Angelicae Sinensis Radix with wine, and stand for a while until completely moistened. Put the drug into a hot stir-frying pot, heat on a gentle fire, keep stir-frying until the surface of the drug become dark yellow, take it out and cool it. Use 10kg of wine for each 100kg of the slices of Angelicae Sinensis Radix.

1.2 Paeoniae Radix Alba (Baishao)

Mix the clean slices of Paeoniae Radix Alba with wine, stand for a while until completely moistened. Put the drug into a hot stir-frying pot, heat on a gentle fire, keep stir-frying until the surface of the drug becomes yellowish, take them out and let it cool. Use 10kg of wine for each 100kg of the slices of Paeoniae Radix Alba.

1.3 Scutellariae Radix (Huangqin)

Mix the clean slices of Scutellariae Radix with wine, and stand for a while until completely moistened. Put the drug into a hot stir-frying pot, heat on a gentle fire, keep stir-frying until the surface of the drug becomes dark yellow, take them out and let it cool. Use 10kg of wine for each 100kg of the Scutellariae Radix.

2. Stir-frying with vinegar

2.1 Genkwa Flos (Yuanhua)

Mix the clean Genkwa Flos with vinegar, and stand for a while until completely moistened. Put the drug into a hot stir-frying pot, stir-fry on a gentle fire until slightly dry, with a gray-brown surface, take them out and allow to cool. Use 30kg of vinegar for each 100kg of the Genkwa Flos.

2.2 Corvallis Rhizoma (Yanhusuo)

Mix the clean slices of Corvallis Rhizoma with vinegar, and stand for a while until completely moistened. Put the drug into a hot stir-frying pot, heat on a gentle fire, keep stir-frying until the surface of the crude drug becomes dark yellow, take them out and allow to cool. Use 20kg of vinegar for each 100kg of the Corvallis Rhizoma.

3. Stir-frying with salt

3.1 Eucommiae Cortex (Duzhong)

Take Eucommiae Cortex shreds or pieces, mix well with salt water, let it cool thoroughly, place in a hot pot, heat gently, stir-fry until the color deepens, there are burnt spots, and the shreds are easily broken. Remove and let it cool. Use 2 kg of salt for each 100kg of the Eucommiae Cortex.

3.2 Phellodendri Chinensis Cortex (Huangbo)

Mix the slivers or pieces of Phellodendri Chinensis Cortex with salt water, and stand for a while until completely moistened. Put the drug into a hot stir-frying pot, heat on a gentle fire, keep stir-frying until the surface charred, take them out and allow to cool. Use 2kg of salt for each 100kg of the Phellodendri Chinensis Cortex.

3.3 Anemarrhenae Rhizoma（Zhimu）

Put the clean slices of Anemarrhenae Rhizoma into a hot stir-frying pot, heat on a gentle fire, keep stir-frying until the surface charred, spray with salt water and stir-frying to dryness. Take them out and allow to cool. Use 2kg of salt for each 100kg of the Anemarrhenae Rhizoma.

4. Stir-frying drug with ginger juice

4.1 Magnoliae Officinalis Cortex（Houpo）

Take Magnoliae officinalis cortex shreds, mix with ginger juice, smother and moisten, wait for the ginger juice to be absorbed, place in a preheated moderate frying container, fry dry over moderate heat, remove and spread out to dry. Use 10kg of ginger for each 100kg of the Magnoliae officinalis cortex.

4.2 Bambusae Caulis In Taenias（Zhuru）

Take the clean Bambusae Caulis In Taenias, add ginger juice and mix well, smother until the ginger juice is absorbed, place in a preheated frying container, fry with moderate heat until light yellow, remove and spread out to dry. Use 10kg of ginger per 100kg of Bambusae Caulis In Taenias.

5. Stir-frying drug with water diluted honey

5.1 Astragali Radix（Huangqi）

Take condensed honey, add the appropriate amount of boiling water dilution, add astragalus slices mixed, slightly smother and place in a preheated frying container, frying with gentle heat until dark yellow and not sticky hands, and then take it out and spread out to dry. Each 100kg Astragali Radix uese 25kg of refined honey.

5.2 Lilii Bulbus（Baihe）

Take the Lilii Bulbus, put them in a preheated moderate frying container, fry with moderate heat until the color deepens, add the appropriate amount of honey diluted with boiling water, quickly stir-fry evenly, frying with moderate heat until slightly yellow, not sticky when removed, and then cool them. Use 5kg of refined honey per 100kg of Lilii Bulbus.

5.3 Eriobotryae Folium（Pipaye）

Take condensed honey, diluted with boiling water, put Eriobotryae Folium and mix well, smother thoroughly, place in a preheated frying container, fry over moderate heat until slightly yellow and not sticky, take out and spread to dry. Use 20kg of refined honey per 100kg of Eriobotryae Folium.

6. Stir-frying drug with oil

Epimedii Folium（Yinyanghuo）

Melt the sheep fat in a pot before adding Epimedii Folium pieces and stir-frying the pieces till its surface color is slightly yellow. Use 20kg sheep fat for each 100kg Epimedii Folium pieces.

◆ Experiment instruction

1. Primary operations and the notes of the operations

1.1 When using the method of mixing adjuvant first and then stir-frying medicine, the adjuvant should be mixed with medicine evenly and moistened until absorbed or permeated into the inner part of the medicine organization before stir-frying.

1.2 When stir-frying with wine, the container should be covered airtight to prevent the rapid evaporation of wine.

1.3 When the salt is dissolved, the amount of water used should be 4-5 times the amount of salt.

1.4 When ginger juice is prepared, the amount of water used is generally 1 : 1 for the final ginger juice and ginger.

1.5 The time of stir-frying with honey can be slightly longer, as far as possible to remove water to avoid mildew, and pay attention to cool after airtight storage.

1.6 If the amount of liquid adjuvant is less and not easy to mix with the drug, it can be first added a proper amount of boiled water dilution to mix the drug better.

1.7 Most of the drug should be heated on a gentle fire and stirred frequently, so that the drug can be evenly heated, then stir-fried to a specified extent.

1.8 If the drug is first fried and then mixed with auxiliary materials, adjuvant should be evenly sprayed on the drug, do not add along the wall of the pot to avoid rapid evaporation of adjuvant.

1.9 In the sizzling, the fire should not be too large, stir-frying frequently, generally fried until nearly dry, the color deepens, you can take it out of the pan to spread.

2. Format of the experimental report

2.1 Purposes

2.2 Principle

2.3 The content of the experiment

2.4 Discussion

3. Considerations after the experiment

3.1 What are the similarities and differences of stir-frying with different liquid adjuvant?

3.2 Why use the method of frying the drug first and then add the auxiliary materials to stir-frying the Anemarrhenae Rhizoma and other drugs?

3.3 How to prepare the adjuvant of stir-frying with honey, ginger juice, salt and fat, respectively?

3.4 Why use the method of frying first and then adding auxiliary ingredients to the concoction for lily?

3.5 Why do we need to use boiling water when diluting honey?

（Edited by De Ji, Changrun Guo and Yalan Zhao）

实验八　当归及其炮制品中水溶性浸出物的含量测定

实验目的 •••

1. 掌握用热浸法测定当归及不同炮制品中水溶性浸出物的含量。

2. 通过测定和比较当归及其炮制品中水溶性浸出物的含量，理解当归炮制的意义。

实验原理 •••

当归为伞形科植物当归 *Angelica sinensis*（Oliv.）Diels 的干燥根。当归具补血活血、调经止痛、润肠通便之功效。用于血虚萎黄，眩晕心悸，月经不调，经闭痛经，虚寒腹痛，肠燥便秘，风湿痹痛，跌扑损伤，痈疽疮疡。酒当归长于活血通经。用于经闭痛经，风湿痹痛，跌扑损伤。

生当归质润，具有润肠通便之效。酒炙后增强活血通经的作用，多用于经闭痛经，风湿痹痛，跌打损伤。本实验采用热浸测定法，对炮制前后当归中水溶性浸出物的含量进行测定，从而说明炮制的意义。

实验器材 •••

1. **仪器**　分析天平，烧杯，锥形瓶，冷凝回流管，蒸发皿等。

2. **药材**　当归，当归炮制品。

实验内容 •••

水溶性浸出物含量测定

（1）水溶性浸出物制备　取供试品约2~4g，精密称定，置100~250mL的锥形瓶中，精密加水50~100mL，密塞，称定重量，静置1小时后，连接回流冷凝管，加热至沸腾，并保持微沸1小时。放冷后，取下锥形瓶，密塞，再称定重量，用水补足减失的重量，摇匀，用干燥滤器滤过，精密量取滤液25mL，置已干燥至恒重的蒸发皿中，在水浴上蒸干后，于105 ℃干燥3小时，置干燥器中冷却30分钟，迅速精密称定重量。除另有规定外，以干燥品计算供试品中水溶性浸出物的含量（%）。

（2）水溶性浸出物的含量（%）测定

$$浸出物（\%）=（M_2-M_0）/ M_1 \times 100\%$$

式中，M_0为蒸发皿重量（g）；M_1为取样重量（g）；M_2为蒸发皿+干燥后水溶性浸出物重量（g）。

实验指导 •••

1. **预习**　水溶性浸出物的含量测定方法还有哪些？

2. **基本操作和操作注意点**　掌握用热浸法测定当归中水溶性浸出物的含量。

3. **实验报告格式**

（1）实验目的

（2）实验原理

（3）含量测定结果

表8-1 水溶性浸出物的含量

样品	水溶性浸出物的含量（%）
生品	
炮制品	

（4）讨论

4. 思考题

（1）当归含哪些主要活性成分？

（2）当归酒炙后水溶性浸出物含量增加，考虑炮制的目的是什么？

（李　飞　曹衡健　赵雅兰）

Experiment 8 The Assay of Water Soluble Extract in the Crude and the Processed Angelicae Sinensis Radix

◆ Experimental purposes

1. To master the assaying method of water-soluble extract in Angelicae Sinensis Radix and its various processed products by Hot dip method.

2. To learn the significant of processing by comparing the contents of water-soluble extract in Angelicae Sinensis Radix with it processed with wine.

◆ Experimental principle

Angelicae Sinensis Radix is the dried root of *Angelica Sinensis* (Oliv.) Diels. With the functions of enriching blood circulation, regulating menstruation, relieving pain, and relaxing bowels, it is used to treat anemia with dizziness and palpitation: menstrual disorder, amenorrhea, dysmenorrhea, constipation, rheumatic arthralgia, traumatic injuries, carbuncle-abscess and sores. After being processed with wine, it can activate blood to promote menstruation and treat amenorrhea, dysmenorrhea, rheumatic arthralgia, traumatic injuries.

◆ Experimental apparatus

1. Instrument

Analytical balance, beaker, conical flask, condensing return line, evaporating dish.

2. Medicinal materials

Angelicae Sinensis Radix, Processed Angelicae Sinensis Radix.

◆ Experimental content

Determination of the content of water-soluble extracts

1.1 Preparation of water-soluble extract

Take about 2-4 g of the sample, precision weighing, placed in 100-250mL of conical bottle, precision 50-100mL of water, dense plug, weighing, standing for 1 hour, connected with the reflux condensing tube, heated to boiling, and keep the micro-boiling for 1 hour. After cooling, remove the conical bottle, plug it, weigh it again, make up for the weight loss with water, shake it well, filter it with a drying filter, take 25mL of filtrate in a precise amount, place it in a dish that has dried to constant weight, dry it on a water bath at 105℃ for 3 hours, cool it in a desiccator for 30 minutes, and quickly weigh it precisely. Unless otherwise specified, the content (%) of water-soluble extracts in the tested products is calculated as dry products.

1.2 Determination of content (%) of water-soluble extract

$$\text{Extract} \ (\%) = (M_2 - M_0) / M_1 \times 100\%$$

Note:

M_0: Pan weight (g); M_1: Sampling weight (g); M_2: Weight of water-soluble extract after evaporation + drying (g).

◆ Experimental instruction

1. Preview

What are the other methods of assaying water-soluble extract?

2. Primary operations and notes of operations

Master the content of water-soluble extract in Angelicae Sinensis by hot immersion method.

3. Format of the experimental report

3.1 Purposes

3.2 Principle

3.3 Results

Table 8-1　Water-soluble extract content

Sample	Water extract content (%)
Raw sample	
Processed sample	

3.4 Discussion

4. Considerations after the experiment

4.1 What are the central ingredients in Angelicae Sinensis Radix?

4.2 The water-soluble content of Angelicae liquor increases after processing. What is the purpose of processing?

（Edited by Fei Li，Hengjian Cao and Yalan Zhao）

实验九 延胡索及其炮制品中生物碱的煎出量分析

实验目的 ●●●

通过对延胡索生品及醋制品水煎液中总生物碱、延胡索乙素和季铵碱的定量分析，比较延胡索炮制前后生物碱煎出量的变化。

实验原理 ●●●

延胡索是罂粟科植物延胡索 *Corydalis yanhusuo* W.T.Wang 的干燥块茎，具有疏肝理气、行气止痛的作用。临床广泛用于治疗各种痛症。延胡索有多种炮制方法，如醋炒、醋蒸、醋煮、酒炒、盐炒等，现常用醋制。

醋，味酸、苦，性温，具散瘀止血、理气止痛的作用，为中药炮制常用液体辅料。中医认为，醋能引药入肝，增强药物疏肝散瘀、止痛的功效，醋制能增强延胡索疏肝止痛的作用。

现代研究表明延胡索主要含生物碱类成分，其中叔胺型生物碱（如延胡索乙素）具有明显的止痛作用，是延胡索止痛的主要成分。醋制过程中，生物碱能与醋酸形成有机盐，使之水溶性增加。因此，炮制后，水煎剂中的总生物碱和延胡索乙素含量都会增加。在缺氧条件下，季铵类生物碱（如去氢延胡索甲素）能显著延长动物存活时间，增加小鼠心肌对 ^{86}Rb 的摄取率，增加小鼠心肌营养性血流量，是治疗冠心病的有效成分。延胡索在醋制过程中，季铵类生物碱的结构因加热而被破坏，因此醋制品中季铵碱的含量明显低于生品。

本实验分别用电位滴定法、高效液相法、分光光度法测定延胡索及其醋制品水煎液中总生物碱、延胡索乙素和季铵类生物碱的含量。

实验器材 ●●●

1. 仪器 万分之一分析天平，十万分之一分析天平，称量瓶，烧杯，量筒，玻璃漏斗，分液漏斗，容量瓶，真空回收装置，水浴锅，锥形瓶，移液管，碱式滴定管，ZD-2型电位滴定计，高效液相色谱仪，布氏漏斗，磁力搅拌器，抽滤瓶，紫外分光光度计等。

2. 药材及试剂 延胡索生、制品，氨水，三氯甲烷，无水硫酸钠，0.01mol/L硫酸，0.02mol/L氢氧化钠，甲基红-溴甲酚绿指示剂，硅胶G，盐酸，甲醇，0.1%磷酸，三乙胺，延胡索乙素标准品，丙酮（AR），雷氏铵盐，滑石粉，定性滤纸，去氢延胡索甲素标准品。

实验内容 ●●●

1. 延胡索炮制前后总生物碱煎出量的测定。
2. 延胡索炮制前后延胡索乙素煎出量的测定。
3. 延胡索炮制前后季铵碱含量的测定。

实验方法 ●●●

1. 延胡索炮制前后总生物碱煎出量的测定

（1）样品制备 精密称取延胡索生品和制品各5g，分别置于500mL烧杯中，用100mL和50mL水分别煎煮两次，每次分别保持微沸20分钟和10分钟，用脱脂棉过滤，合并滤液，加氨水调至pH10以上，将滤液移至250mL分液漏斗中，分别用20mL三氯甲烷萃取两次，合并萃取液，加10mL蒸馏水洗涤1次，加入5g无水硫酸钠脱水后，过滤，挥干三氯甲烷，得残渣，即为总生物碱。

（2）含量测定　精密吸取0.01mol/L硫酸15mL溶解总生物碱，用0.02mol/L氢氧化钠滴定，以电位测定法指示终点，等当点为pH5.1（或加甲基红–溴甲酚绿指示剂2滴，终点颜色由红变绿）。

（3）计算（按延胡索乙素计算）

$$含量\% = \frac{C_{H_2SO_4} \cdot V_{H_2SO_4} \cdot 2 - C_{NaOH} \cdot V_{NaOH}}{W} \times 355.4 \times 100\%$$

式中，W为延胡索重量（g）。

2. 延胡索炮制前后延胡索乙素的煎出量的测定

（1）色谱条件与系统适应性试验　以十八烷基硅烷键合硅胶为填充剂，以甲醇–0.1%磷酸溶液（三乙胺调pH6.0）（55∶45）为流动相，检测波长为280nm。理论塔板数按延胡索乙素计算应不低于3000。

（2）对照品溶液的制备　精密称取延胡索乙素对照品适量，加甲醇制成每1mL含46μg的溶液，即得。

（3）供试品溶液的制备　除将"加氨水调pH10以上"改为"加盐酸调至pH 6~7"外，其余同总碱测定。

（4）标准曲线的制备　将对照品溶液按照不同比例进行稀释，精密吸取各不同稀释倍数的对照品溶液各10μL，注入液相色谱仪，按照标准曲线的测定方法，进行测定，制备标准曲线。

（5）样品测定　分别精密吸取对照品溶液与供试品溶液各10μL，注入液相色谱仪，测定，即得。

$$含量\% = \frac{C \times 10}{W \times 10^6} \times 100\%$$

式中，C为所测得的样品浓度（μg/mL）；W为取样量（g）。

3. 延胡索炮制前后季铵碱含量的测定

（1）标准曲线制备　取去氢延胡索甲素对照品溶于盐酸酸化的水溶液（pH 2~3）中，加过量新鲜配制的2%雷氏铵盐溶液，待完全沉淀后，抽滤，沉淀用盐酸酸化的微酸性水溶液（pH 5~6）冲洗，至无雷氏铵盐，然后置干燥器中常温真空干燥。精密称取以上得到的去氢延胡索甲素雷氏复盐200mg，置50mL容量瓶中，用盐酸酸化的丙酮（pH 2~3）溶解，并稀释至刻度。精取上述溶液2.0mL、4.0mL、6.0mL、8.0mL、10.0mL，分别置于10mL容量瓶中，用酸性丙酮（pH 2~3）稀释至刻度，于721型分光光度计525nm处测定吸收度，以酸性丙酮（pH 2~3）为空白对照，以去氢延胡索甲素雷氏复盐的浓度为横坐标，吸收度为纵坐标，绘制标准曲线。

（2）样品液的制备　精密称取延胡索生品和制品各10g，分别置于500mL烧杯中，用200mL和100mL水分别煎煮两次，每次保持微沸20分钟，用脱脂棉过滤，合并滤液，加盐酸调至pH 2~3，滴加新鲜配制的2%雷氏铵盐至无沉淀产生，用磁力搅拌器搅拌30分钟，使其充分沉淀，然后于冰箱中放置30分钟，沉淀用布氏漏斗抽滤，先用冰水洗去雷氏铵盐，再用酸性丙酮洗至沉淀全部溶出，定容于50mL容量瓶中，备用。

（3）样品液测定　将上述样品液在721型分光光度计525nm处测定吸收值。

（4）计算

$$季铵碱\% = \frac{C \times 50}{W \times 1000} \times 100\%$$

式中，C为样品吸收值在标准曲线上相对应的浓度（mg/mL）；W为取样量（g）。

实验指导 •••

1. 基本操作和操作注意点

（1）应事先检查分液漏斗和滴定管是否漏液。

（2）延胡索水煎液中有较多的黏液，不好过滤，可加脱脂棉过滤。

（3）调pH要准确，否则测定结果会受到影响。

（4）三氯甲烷萃取要完全，以少量多次为佳；若三氯甲烷层乳化，可用玻棒搅拌助其分层。

（5）用酸性丙酮洗脱季铵碱雷氏复盐时，应洗脱完全。

2. 实验报告格式

（1）实验目的

（2）实验原理

（3）实验内容

（4）讨论

① 总生物碱含量

表9-1 总生物碱含量

样品	重量（g）	消耗NaOH（mL）	总碱百分含量（%）
生品			
炮制品			

② 延胡索乙素含量

表9-2 延胡索乙素含量

样品	重量（g）	As	AR	百分含量（%）
生品				
炮制品				

③ 季铵碱含量

表9-3 季铵碱含量

样品	重量（g）	吸收度（A）	百分含量（%）
生品			
炮制品			

3. 实验后思考

（1）通过对延胡索生品及醋制品水煎液中总生物碱和季铵碱含量变化的比较，能得到什么结论？

（2）延胡索中生物碱的含量测定，除了本实验中提到的方法外，还有哪些方法？

（徐　健　赵雅兰）

Experiment 9   The Assay of Alkaloids in the Crude and the Processed Corydalis Rhizoma

◆ Experimental purpose

To compare the contents of total alkaloids, *dl*-tetrahydropalmatine and dehydrocorydaline in the water decoction between the crude Corydalis Rhizoma and the processed one.

◆ Experimental principle

Corydalis Rhizoma, also called *Yuanhu*, is the dried tuber of *Corydalis yanhusuo* W.T.Wang. (*Fam. Papaveraceae*). It can sooth the liver and regulate the flow of Qi, and also promote the flow of Qi and relieve the pain. According to the traditional Chinese medicine (TCM), it is used widely to relieve most kinds of pains. There are many processing methods of Corydalis Rhizoma, such as stir-frying, steaming and boiling with vinegar, stir-frying with wine, salt, and so on. Now it is usually processed with vinegar.

Vinegar, which tastes sour and bitter in flavor and warm in nature. It can remove the blood stasis, stop bleeding and relieve the pain. It is usually used as liquid subsidiary material. According to the TCM, vinegar can draw the drug into the liver, strengthen the drug's function of soothing the liver, removing the blood stasis and relieving the pain. The processing with vinegar can enhance Corydalis Rhizoma's function of the soothing the liver and relieving paining.

According to the modern reports, Corydalis Rhizoma mainly contains alkaloids, especially the tertiary amine type alkaloids (such as *dl*–tetrahydropalmatine), which have the obvious function of relieving pain and is the main constituent of pain relief. After being processed with vinegar, the acetic acid can form organic salts with alkaloids to increase the water solubility. Therefore, the content of the total alkaloids and *dl*-tetrahydropalmatine is both increased in the water decoction. As the result, the analgesic effect is increased.

In the endurance test of the oxygen deficiency, the quaternary amine type alkaloids (such as dehydrocorydaline) can significantly prolong the animal living span and increase the absorbance on ^{86}Rb of the mice's myocardium (cardiac muscle). It also can increase nutritional blood vessel (or blood circulation) and is the effective constituent of treating coronary heart disease.

After being processed with vinegar, the structure of the quaternary ammonium alkaloids is destroyed by heating. Therefore, the content of quaternary amine type alkaloids in vinegar products is significantly lower than that in crude products.

In our experiments, the contents of total alkaloids, *dl*-tetrahydropalmatine and the quaternary amine type alkaloids are determinated by potentiometric titration, HPLC, spectrophotometric methods respectively to compare the difference between the processed and the crude drug.

◆ Experimental apparatus

1. Instruments

Analytical balance (1/10000, 1/100000), weighing bottle, beaker, graduated cylinder, glass funnel, separate funnel, volumetric flask, vacuum recovery apparatus, water bath, conical flask pipe, transfer pipet, basic buret（burette）, ZD-2 type potentiometric titrator, chromatography jar, thin layer plate, micro-syringe, electric drier, HPLC, Buchner funnel, magnetic agitator（stirrer）, suction flask, UV spectrophotometer.

2. Medicinal materials and chemicals

The crude Corydalis Rhizoma and the processed one, Ammonium hydroxide, chloroform, sodium sulfate anhydrous, 0.01mol/L sulfuric acid, 0.02mol/L sodium hydroxide, methylred-Bromocresol green indicator, silica gel G, hydrochloric acid, methanol, 0.1% phosphoric acid, triethylamine, *dl*-tetrahydropalmatine, （standard reference material, SRM）, acetone, Ammonium reineckate, talcum powder, qualitative filter paper, dehydrocorydaline（SRM）.

◆ Experimental content

1. Determination of the total alkaloids.

2. Determination of *dl*-tetrahydropalmatine with HPLC.

3. Determination the amount of the quaternary amine type alkaloids.

◆ Experimental methods

1. Determination of the total alkaloids

1.1 The preparation of the samples: Weigh precisely 5g of the crude drug and the processed drug, put them into two 500mL beakers respectively, then add 100mL and 50mL water to boil it for two times. Each time the decoction should keep slightly boilintg for 20 minutes and 10 minutes then filter the decoction with absorbent cotton and mix the filtrate respectively. Add the ammonium hydroxide to adjust pH value of each filtrate until above 10, then transfer each filtrate to 250mL separating funnel, and then extract it with 20mL chloroform twice until showed negative reaction with alkaloid reagents, collect the exaction and wash with 10mL distilled water, adding 5 g sodium sulfate anhydrous to dehydration and volatilizing chloroform.

1.2 Determination: Precise suction of 15mL 0.0lmol/L sulfuric acid. Titrate with 0.02mol/L sodium hydroxide by indicating end with potentiometer titration, the equivalence point is pH 5.1（or add two drops of methyl red and Bromocresol green indicator, the end is indicated by the color changing from red into green）.

1.3 Calculation（calculated by *dl*-tetrahydropalmatine）

$$\text{Content }\%=\frac{C_{\text{H}_2\text{SO}_4}\cdot V_{\text{H}_2\text{SO}_4}\cdot2-C_{\text{NaOH}}\cdot V_{\text{NaOH}}}{W}\times355.4\times100\%$$

Note:

W: the weight of sample（g）.

2. Determination of *dl*-tetrahydropalmatine with HPLC

2.1 Chromatographic system and system suitability: Use octadecylsilane bonded silica gel as the stationary phase and methanol -1% phosphoric acid（55：45）as the mobile phase（using triethylamine to adjust pH to 6.0）. The wavelength of the detector is 280 nm. The number of theoretical plates of the column is not less than 3000, calculated with the reference of the peak of *dl*-tetrahydropalmatine.

2.2 Preparation of the reference solution: Weigh accurately proper amount of *dl*-tetrahydropalmatine（SRM） and add methanol to make reference solution at the concentration of 46 μg/mL.

2.3 Preparation of the test solution: Add hydrochloric acid to adjust pH to 6-7 instead of adding ammonium hydroxide to adjust pH above 10. The other steps are as the same as the determination of total alkaloids.

2.4 Preparation of the standard curve: Dilute the reference solution into different concentration at a certain rate. Inject accurately 10μL above diluted solution into HPLC. Determinate by the method of standard curve and draw the standard curve.

2.5 Determination of samples: Inject 10μL of reference solution and test solution to the HPLC respectively and determinate.

$$dl\text{-tetrahydropalmatine }\% = \frac{C \times 10}{W \times 10^6} \times 100\%$$

Note:

C: the content of test solution (μg/mL); W: the weight of sample (g).

3. Determination the amount of the quaternary amine type alkaloids

3.1 Preparation of the standard curve: Take the dehydrocorydaline solution, (acidified by hydrochloric acid to pH 2-3), add adequate fresh prepared 2% Ammonium reineckate to make the dehydrocorydaline precipitate completely, then filter it under reduced pressure. The precipitation is washed with slightly acid water (acidified by hydrochloric acid to pH 5-6) until the rinsing water has no ammonium reineckate. Then transfer the precipitation in the desiccator under vacuum and dry at the room temperature.

And weigh 200mg above dried double salt (dehydrocorydaline and ammonium reineckate) precisely, put it into a 50mL volumetric flask, dissolve with acetone (acidified by hydrochloric acid to pH 2-3), and dilute it to the scale.

Transfer above solution 2.0, 4.0, 6.0, 8.0, 10.0mL precisely to 10mL volumetric flask respectively, and dilute them to the scale with acidified acetone (pH 2-3) then determine the absorbance at 525nm with 721 type spectrophotometer.

The blank control sample is the acidified acetone (pH 2-3), then draw the standard curve to make the concentration of the double salt as X-coordinate and make the absorbance as Y-coordinate.

3.2 Preparation of the sample: Weigh precisely 10g both the crude drug and the processed drug and put them into two 500mL beakers respectively, then add 200mL and 100mL water to decoct the drug for two times, each time the decoction should keep slightly boiling for 20 minutes. Filter the decoction with absorbent cotton and mix the filtrate respectively, and add the hydrochloric acid to adjust the acid degree to pH 2-3, dropping the fresh prepared 2% ammonium reineckate to above solution until no more precipitate produced. Then stir them with magnetic agitator for 30 minutes, to make it precipitate adequately, then keep it in refrigerator for 30 min, and the precipitate is filtered under reduced pressure by Buchner funnel (talcum powder used as filter aid), wash the ammonium reineckate off the precipitate with water, then dissolve the total precipitate with acidified acetone, and transfer the acetone to 50mL volumetric flask, add the acidified acetone to the scale.

3.3 Determination of the sample: Determinate the absorbance of above solution at 525nm with spectrophotometer.

3.4 Calculation:

$$\text{The quaternary amine type alkaloids }\% = \frac{C \times 50}{W \times 1000} \times 100\%$$

Note:

C: the concentration of the sample (mg/mL); W: the weight of sample (g).

◆ Experimental instruction

1 Primary operations and notes of operations

1.1 To check whether the separatory funnel and basic buret leaking solution before use.

1.2 The water decoction of Corydalis Rhizoma is not easy to filtrate due to it has much starch, so we can deal it with absorbent cotton.

1.3 Adjust the pH value accurately. Otherwise, the results of the determination will be influenced.

1 4 The extraction by chloroform should be adequately. It is better according to "the smaller amount, the more times". If the emulsified layer appeared during the extraction by chloroform, we could use the glass rod stir it slightly to make the lay separate.

1.5 When washing quaternary ammonium reineckate using acidic actone, it should be washed thoroughly.

2. Format of the experimental report

2.1 Purpose of the experiment

2.2 Principle of the experiment

2.3 Content and results of the experiment

2.4 Discussion

2.4.1 The total alkaloids amount

Table 9-1 Total alkaloids amount

Sample	Weight(g)	Volume of NaOH(mL)	Content(%)
Crude drug			
Processed drug			

2.4.2 The *dl*-tetrahydropalmatine amount

Table 9-2 *dl*-tetrahydropalmatine amount

Sample	Weight(g)	As	AR	Content(%)
Crude drug				
Processed drug				

2.4.3 The quaternary amine type alkaloids amount

Table 9-3 Quaternary amine type alkaloids amount

Sample	Weight(g)	Absorbance(A)	Content(%)
Crude drug			
Processed drug			

3. Considerations after the experiment

3.1 After comparing the alkaloids amount and the quaternary amine type alkaloids amount between the crude drug and processed drug, what can you conclude according to the variation?

3.2 What other methods are there to determine the alkaloid besides those mentioned in this experiment?

(Edited by Jian Xu and Yalan Zhao)

实验十　麻黄蜜炙前后发汗、平喘作用的比较

实验目的 ●●●

通过比较麻黄蜜炙前后发汗作用和止咳平喘作用的变化，理解麻黄蜜炙的炮制原理。

实验原理 ●●●

麻黄包括草麻黄 *Ephedra sinica* Stapf.、木贼麻黄 *E. equisetina* Bge. 和中麻黄 *E. intermedia* Schrenk et C. A. Mey.，是一种常用中药，具有发汗散寒、宣肺平喘、利水消肿的功效。它含有多种生物碱，主要含 *l*-麻黄碱（*l*-ephedrine，又称麻黄素）和 *d*-伪麻黄碱（*d*-pseudoephedrine，又称异麻黄素），另含有挥发油。麻黄碱能松弛支气管平滑肌，有平喘作用；挥发油能抑制流感病毒，并能兴奋汗腺，有发汗作用；油中 L-α-萜品烯醇及 2,3,5,6-四甲基吡嗪具有平喘作用。

传统经验认为麻黄经蜜炙后发汗作用降低，平喘作用增强，现代化学研究证实麻黄蜜炙后生物碱减少甚微，而挥发油含量虽然减少二分之一左右，但是在其油的组成中具有平喘作用 L-α-萜品烯醇、四甲基吡嗪、石竹烯、芳樟醇相对含量均增高，从而增强平喘作用，减少了发汗作用。

本实验围绕麻黄炮制前后发汗平喘药理作用的比较进行研究。

实验器材 ●●●

1. 仪器　显微镜，水浴锅，电子天平，超声雾化器。

2. 药材及试剂　麻黄药材，甲醛，乙醇，二甲苯，石蜡，碘，可溶性淀粉，和田-高垣试剂，无水乙醇，蓖麻油和氯化乙酰胆碱。

3. 实验动物　健康昆明种小鼠，体重18~22g，雌雄各半；豚鼠，体重150~200g，雌雄各半。

实验内容 ●●●

1. 麻黄蜜炙前后对小鼠发汗作用的比较。

2. 麻黄蜜炙前后对动物平喘作用的比较。

实验方法 ●●●

1. 供试液制备　精密称取麻黄生品和蜜炙品各10g，各加10倍量水浸泡20分钟，煎煮30分钟后，去沫，过滤，滤液另存，滤渣继续加8倍量水煎煮30分钟，过滤。合并滤液，浓缩至1g/mL，备用。

2. 麻黄蜜炙前后对小鼠发汗作用的比较

（1）将小鼠随机分组（空白对照组、麻黄生品组、麻黄蜜炙组），每组10只，给药前禁食12小时，用棉签蘸取无水乙醇轻轻将足趾部污染擦洗干净，每只按10mL/kg剂量灌胃给药，空白对照组给予相同体积的生理盐水。将小鼠分别固定，仰位固定，暴露双后肢。给药后30分钟将大鼠足趾部皮肤涂上和田-高垣试剂A（取碘2g溶于100mL无水乙醇），待充分干燥后，再薄薄涂上B液（取可溶性淀粉50g，蓖麻油100mL，两者混合），用放大镜仔细观察着色点颜色和数量，每10分钟记录1次，持续观察30分钟。

（2）应用SPSS 10.0软件对实验结果进行统计学处理，计量资料均采用 $\bar{X} \pm S$ 表示，两组间比较采用 t 检验，多组均数比较采用方差分析。

3. 麻黄蜜炙前后对动物平喘作用的比较

（1）将豚鼠放入密闭玻璃钟罩内，以超声喷雾器定量喷雾4%氯化乙酰胆碱液，每只豚鼠接受喷雾量6mL，5秒后立即取出，记录豚鼠从接受喷雾开始到出现喘息性抽搐跌倒的潜伏期，引喘潜伏期大于120秒的舍弃，合格豚鼠随机分组（麻黄生品组，麻黄蜜炙品组，空白对照组），每组10只，给药前禁食12小时，每只按10mL/kg剂量灌胃给药，给药后1小时将豚鼠放入喷雾装置内，以4%氯化乙酰胆碱定量恒压喷雾5秒，分别记录麻黄生品和蜜炙品的豚鼠引喘潜伏期。

（2）应用SPSS 10.0软件对实验结果讲行统计学处理，计量资料均采用$X \pm S$表示，两组问比较采用t检验，多组均数比较采用方差分析。

实验指导 •••

1. 基本操作和操作注意点

（1）基本操作　掌握发汗、平喘药理实验操作方法。

（2）操作注意事项　①药材一定要拣去杂质方可称重。②称量小鼠体重前，要擦干小鼠的汗液，否则会影响实验结果。③进行超声喷雾器定量恒压喷雾时，要注意自我防护。

2. 实验报告格式

（1）实验目的

（2）实验原理

（3）实验数据及计算结果

（4）讨论

3. 实验后思考

通过比较麻黄蜜炙前后发汗量、汗腺导管内径大小和引喘潜伏期的测定结果，说明麻黄蜜炙的目的和意义。

（徐　健　赵雅兰）

Experiment 10　Comparative Study on the Effects of Inducing Perspiration and Relieving Asthma on the Crude and Ephedrae Herba Processed with Honey

◆ Experimental purpose

To learn the purpose and meanings of processing through the comparative study on the effects of inducing perspiration and relieving asthma on Ephedrae Herba before and after stir-frying with honey.

◆ Experimental principle

Ephedrae Herba includes *Ephedra sinica* Stapf., *Ephedra intermedia* Schrenk et C.A.Mey. and *Ephedra equisetina* Bge. It is a TCM often used, which has the function of inducing perspiration for dispelling cold to relieve asthma and to cause diuresis. Herb Ephedrae contains many kinds of alkaloids including *l*-ephedrine, *d*-pseudoephedrine and volatile oil. Ephedrine can slack the smooth muscles of bronchus and has the function of relieving asthma. Volatile oil can resist the influenza virus and stimulate the sweat gland and has the function of inducing perspiration. L-α-terpineol and 2,3,5,6-tetramethyl-pyrazine contained in the volatile oil have the action of relieving asthma.

Traditional experience considers that after being processed with honey, the Ephedrae Herba's action of inducing perspiration of processed with honey is decreased, whereas the function of relieving asthma is increased. Modern chemical research has proved that the content of alkaloids of Ephedrae Herba processed with honey is decreased slightly although the content of volatile oil is decreased by half. However, the relative contents of L-α-terpineol, 2,3,5,6-tetramethyl-pyrazine, caryophyllene, limonen and linalool having the action of resisting bacteria and virus, promoting expectoration, relieving a cough increase, which can improve the function of relieving asthma but decrease the function of inducing perspiration.

This experiment studies the differences on the effects of inducing perspiration and relieving asthma on Ephedrae Herba before and after stir-frying with honey.

◆ Experimental apparatus

1. Instruments

Microscope, water bath, electronic scales, ultrasonic atomizer.

2. Medicinal materials and Chemicals

Ephedrae Herba, formaldehyde, ethanol, xylene, paraffin, Acetylcholine chloride, castor-oil, iodine, soluble starch, anhydrous ethanol.

3. Animals

Healthy Kunming mice, weighting 18-22g, half male and half female; Guinea pig, weighting 150-200g, half male and half female.

◆ Experimental content

1. Comparing of inducing perspiration effect of crude and processed drugs.
2. Comparing of relieving asthma effect of crude and processed drugs.

◆ Experimental methods

1. Preparation of test solution

Weigh accurately 10g crude and processed Ephedrae Herba respectively. Add 100mL water and infuse for 20 minutes. Decoct for 30 minutes, filter, combine the filtrate. Add 8 times the amount of water to the filter residue and cook for 30 minutes. Combine the filtrate to the concentration of 1g/mL as test solution.

2. Comparing of inducing perspiration effect of crude and processed drug

2.1 The qualified rats are divided into three groups randomly (crude drug group, processed group and blank group), ten rats for each group. The rats are fastened for 12 hours before administration. The drug is given to the rats at the dose of 10mL/kg by intragastric administration while equal volume of physiological saline for blank group. Clean the rats' toes with cotton balls dipped in the ethanol. Fix the rats supinely exposing the hindlimbs. 30 minutes after administration, the skin of toes is smeared with reagent A (dissolve 2g of iodine with ethanol), let it dry completely and then apply the reagent B (mix 50g of soluble starch and 100mL of castor oil). Observe the color and amount of colored point using magnifying glass for 30 minutes and record the results every 10 minutes.

2.2 All the data are analyzed using SPSS version 10.0 software and expressed as $X \pm S$. The t-test is used for comparison between the two groups, and the analysis of variance is used for mean comparison between multiple groups.

3. Comparing of relieving asthma effect of crude and processed drug

3.1 Put the guinea pigs in a closed glass bell jar, an ultrasonic nebulizer is used to quantitatively spray vapor of acetylcholine chloride. 6mL vapor for each guinea pig, and take it out after 5 seconds. Record the latent period from the beginning of spraying to the asthmatic convulsion and fall down. If the time is longer than 120 seconds, the value is abandoned. The qualified guinea pigs are divided into three groups randomly (crude drug group, processed group and blank group), ten guinea pigs for each group. The guinea pigs are fastened for 12 hours before administration. The drug is given to the guinea pigs at the dose of 10mL/kg by intragastric administration. And 1 hour later, they are put into the closed glass bell jar, spraying 4% acetylcholine chloride for 5 seconds, record the latent period of asthmatic convulsion.

3.2 All the data are analyzed using SPSS version 10.0 software and expressed as $X \pm S$. The t-test was used for comparison between the two groups, and the analysis of variance was used for mean comparison between multiple groups.

◆ Experimental instruction

1. Primary operations and the notes of operations

1.1 Primary operations

Master the operational methods of sweating and asthma relieving pharmacological experiments.

1.2 Notes of operations

1.2.1 Foreign matters must be eliminated before weighing.

1.2.2 Before weighing the mice, the sweat of the mice should be wiped dry, otherwise it will affect the experimental results.

1.2.3 When conducting ultrasonic sprayer quantitative constant pressure spray, pay attention to self-protection.

2. Format of experimental report

2.1 Purpose

2.2 Principle

2.3 Experimental data and calculating results

2.4 Discussion

3. Considerations after the experiment

By comparing the measurement results of sweating volume, inner diameter of sweat gland ducts, and incubation period for inducing asthma after processing Ephedrae Herba, the purpose and significance of ephedra honey roasting are explained.

（Edited by Jian Xu and Yalan Zhao）

实验十一 淫羊藿及炮制品中总黄酮和淫羊藿苷的测定

实验目的 ●●●

掌握淫羊藿总黄酮和淫羊藿苷的含量测定方法。

实验原理 ●●●

淫羊藿为小檗科植物淫羊藿 *Epimedium brevicornum* Maxim.、箭叶淫羊藿 *Epimedium sagittatum*（Sieb.et Zucc.）Maxim.、柔毛淫羊藿 *Epimedium pubescens* Maxim.或朝鲜淫羊藿 *Epimedium koreanum* Nakai 的干燥叶。其性味辛热，入肾经。具有温肾壮阳，祛风湿的功效。中医临床用于阳痿，腰膝酸软和高血压等病证的治疗。临床上多使用其炮制品——羊脂油炙品。长期的临床实践证明：羊脂油炙可增强淫羊藿的功效。

现代科学研究表明，黄酮类成分如淫羊藿苷（Icariin）是淫羊藿的主要活性成分。因此，本实验通过比较淫羊藿及其炮制品中总黄酮和淫羊藿苷的含量，说明其炮制的作用。

实验器材 ●●●

1. 仪器 超声仪，紫外分光光度计，50mL具塞锥形瓶，20mL移液管，玻璃漏斗，25mL容量瓶，0.5mL、1mL、2mL、5mL移液管分析天平，液相色谱仪。

2. 药材及试剂 淫羊藿（生品），淫羊藿苷对照品，乙醇，滤纸，称量纸。

实验内容 ●●●

1. 总黄酮含量测定

（1）标准曲线的制备 精密称取淫羊藿苷对照品4mg置于25mL容量瓶中，用50%乙醇溶解并稀释至刻度。分别从中精密吸取0.5mL、1.0mL、1.5mL、2.0mL、2.5mL，置于25mL容量瓶中，定容至刻度。于紫外分光光度计270nm处，以50%乙醇为空白对照，分别测定吸收度，并以吸收度为纵坐标，淫羊藿苷浓度为横坐标绘制标准曲线。

（2）样品的测定 分别称取淫羊藿及炙淫羊藿0.2g，置50mL具塞锥形瓶中，精密加入50%乙醇20mL，超声提取40分钟，提取2次，滤纸过滤至50mL容量瓶中，残渣用少量50%乙醇洗涤，并用50%乙醇稀释至刻度。精密吸取上述溶液2mL置25mL容量瓶中，用50%乙醇稀释并定容至刻度，于270nm处测定吸收度，并参照标准曲线计算被测样品的浓度。

$$含量（\%）=\frac{C \times 50 \times 25 \times 10^{-3} \times 100}{2 \times W}\%$$

式中，C为样品中总黄酮浓度（mg/mL）；W为样品重量（g）。

2. 总黄酮醇苷含量测定

（1）色谱条件与系统适用性试验 十八烷基硅烷键合硅胶为填充剂（柱长为250mm，内径为4.6mm）；以乙腈为流动相A，水为流动相B，按表11-1中的规定进行梯度洗脱；柱温为30℃；检测波长为270nm。理论板数按淫羊藿苷峰计算应不低于8000。

表11-1 梯度洗脱程序

时间（分钟）	流动相A（%）	流动相B（%）
0～30	24→26	76→74
30～31	26→45	74→55
31～45	45→47	55→53

（2）对照品溶液的制备 取淫羊藿苷对照品适量，精密称定，加甲醇制成每1mL含40μg的溶液，即得。

（3）供试品溶液的制备 取本品叶片，粉碎过三号筛，取约0.2g，精密称定，置具塞锥形瓶中，精密加入稀乙醇20mL，称定重量，超声处理（功率400W，频率50kHz）1小时，放冷，再称定重量，用稀乙醇补足减失的重量，摇匀，滤过，取续滤液，即得。

（4）测定法 精密吸取对照品溶液与供试品溶液各10μL，注入液相色谱仪，测定。以淫羊藿苷对照品为参照，以其相应的峰为S峰，计算朝藿定A、朝藿定B、朝藿定C峰的相对保留时间，其相对保留时间应在规定值的±5%范围之内。相对保留时间及校正因子见表11-2。

表11-2 相对保留时间及校正因子

待测成分（峰）	相对保留时间	校正因子
朝藿定A	0.73	1.35
朝藿定B	0.81	1.28
朝藿定C	0.90	1.22
淫羊藿苷（S）	1.00	1.00

以淫羊藿苷对照品为对照，分别乘以校正因子，计算朝藿定A、朝藿定B、朝藿定C和淫羊藿苷的含量。

实验指导

1. 基本操作和操作注意点

（1）掌握淫羊藿中总黄酮和总黄酮醇苷的含量测定方法。

（2）紫外分光光度计应预热稳定后方可测定。

2. 实验报告格式

（1）实验目的

（2）实验原理

（3）实验内容及计算结果

①总黄酮醇苷含量测定

表11-3 淫羊藿炮制前后总黄酮的含量

样品	重量（g）	吸收度（A）	浓度（μg/mL）	百分含量（%）
生品				
炙品				

②淫羊藿苷含量测定

表11-4　淫羊藿炮制前后总黄酮醇苷的含量

样品	重量（g）	浓度（μg/mL）	百分含量（%）
生品			
炙品			

（4）讨论

3. 实验后思考

（1）淫羊藿中总黄酮的药理作用是什么？

（2）黄酮类化合物的含量测定方法还有哪些？

（郭常润　赵雅兰）

Experiment 11   The Assay of the Total Flavonoes and Icariin in the Crude and the Processed Epimedii Folium

◆ Experimental purpose

To master the quantitative determination method of total flavones and Icariin in Epimedii Folium and its processed drug.

◆ Experimental principle

Epimedii Folium consists of the dried aerial parts of *Epimedium brevicornum* Maxim., *Epimedium sagittatum* (Sieb.et Zucc.) Maxim., *Epimedium pubescens* Maxim.and *Epimedium koreanum* Nakai. It is pungent and hot. Its functions are to warm up the kidney, to strengthen Yang and to dispel cold and dampness. It is used to reinforce vital function of the sexual organ for the treatment of impotence, aching back and knees with cold intolerance and climacteric hypertension. It is commonly processed with sheep fat, which has been proved through long clinic practice to strengthen the functions of Epimedii Folium.

Modern scientific research has proved that the flavones in Epimedii Folium such as Icariin are main active components.

This experiment determines the content of flavones and Icariin in Epimedii Folium and its processed product, so as to understand why the drug should be processed with sheep fat.

◆ Experimental apparatus

1. Instruments

Ultraviolet photometer, 50mL conic bottle, 25mL volumetric bottle, 0.5mL, 1.0mL, 2.0mL, 5.0mL and 20.0mL gauge glass, glass filter, filter paper.

2. Medicinal materials and chemicals

Epimedii Folium, Icariin, alcohol, filter paper and weighing paper.

◆ Experimental content

1. Determination of total flavones in Epimedii Folium

1.1 Preparation of standard curve; Weigh accurately 4mg Icariin into a 25mL volumetric flask and dissolve with 50% alcohol solution. Transfer accurately 0.5, 1.0, 1.5, 2.0 and 2.5mL the above solution respectively into five 25mL volumetric bottles, add 25mL 50% alcohol solution to the scale. The absorbance of the resulting solutions is separately determined in ultraviolet photometer with the wavelength of 270nm and 50% alcohol solution as a comparative solution.

1.2 Sample determination: Weigh accurately 0.2g of Epimedii Folium pieces and sheep fat-processed product separately into two 50mL conic bottles and extracted with accurate 20mL of 50% alcohol solution under supersonic for 40 minutes twice. The extraction solutions are filtered into 50mL volumetric bottles, adding 50% alcohol solution to the scale. Transfer 2.0mL of the above solutions are separately to 25mL volumetric bottles and diluted with 50% alcohol solution to the scale. The absorbance is separately determined in ultraviolet photometer at the wavelength of 270nm and 50% alcohol solution as a comparative solution. The content of the flavones in

Epimedii Folium pieces and the sheep-processed drug are calculated in accordance with the standard curve.

$$\text{Content}\ (\%) = \frac{C \times 50 \times 25 \times 10^{-3} \times 100}{2 \times W}\%$$

Note：

C：the concentration of the flavones (mg/mL)；W：the weight of the samples (g) .

2. Assay of total flavonol glycosides in Epimedii Folium

2.1 Chromatographic conditions and system suitability test：octadecylsilane bonded silica gel as filler (column length 250mm, inner diameter 4.6mm)；acetonitrile as mobile phase A, water as mobile phase B, gradient elution according to the following table；column temperature 30℃ ; detection wavelength 270nm. theoretical plate number should be not less than 8000 according to the peak of Epimedium.

Table 11-1 Gradient elution procedure

Time (minutes)	Mobile phase A (%)	Mobile phase B (%)
0 ~ 30	24→26	76→74
30 ~ 31	26→45	74→55
31 ~ 45	45→47	55→53

2.2 Preparation of control solution：Take an appropriate amount of Epimedium control, weigh precisely, add methanol to make a solution containing 40μg per 1mL.

2.3 Preparation of the test solution：Take the leaf of the product, crush it and pass it through No.3 sieve, take about 0.2g, weigh it precisely, put it in a conical flask with stopper, add 20mL of dilute ethanol precisely, weigh it, ultrasonic treatment (power 400W, frequency 50kHz) for 1 hour, let it cool, weigh it again, make up the lost weight with dilute ethanol, shake it well, filter it, take the filtrate and obtain it.

2.4 Determination method：Take 10μL of the control solution and 10μL of the test solution, inject them into the liquid chromatograph and determine. The relative retention times of the peaks of patchouli A, B and C should be within ± 5% of the specified values. The relative retention time and correction factor are shown in the following table.

Table 11-2 Relative retention time and correction factor

Component to be measured (peak)	Relative retention time	Correction factor
Epimedin A	0. 73	1. 35
Epimedin B	0. 81	1. 28
Epimedin C	0. 90	1. 22
Icariin（S）	1. 00	1. 00

The contents of Epimedin A, B, C and Icariin are calculated by multiplying the correction factors with Icariin × control as the control, respectively.

◆ Experimental instruction

1. Primary operations and notes of the operations

1.1 Master the quantitative determination method of flavones and icariin in Epimedii Folium and its processed drug.

1.2 Ultraviolet photometer should be preheated and stable before measurement .

2. Format of the experimental report

2.1 Purpose

2.2 Principle

2.3 Experimental data and calculating results

Table 11-3　Content of flavones

Sample	Weight (g)	Absorbance (A)	Concentration (μg/mL)	Content (%)
Epimedii Folium				
Processed drug				

Table 11-4　Content of total flavonol glycosides

Sample	Weight (g)	Concentration (μg/mL)	Content (%)
Epimedii Folium			
Processed drug			

2.4 Discussion

3. Considerations after the experiment

3.1 What are the pharmacological functions of flavones in Epimedii Folium?

3.2 What are the other quantitative determination methods of flavones besides photometric method?

（ Edited by Changrun Guo and Yalan Zhao ）

第四章 煅 法

实验十二 煅法的代表药物炮制

实验目的 •••

1. 掌握各种煅法的操作方法、基本要求。
2. 熟悉煅法的分类。
3. 了解煅法的目的。

实验原理 •••

将药物进行高温煅烧的炮制方法称之为煅法。根据药物的性质和煅制方法及要求分为明煅法、煅淬法、闷煅（扣锅煅）法。

将药物直接置于无烟炉或耐火容器中煅烧（不隔绝空气），使药物酥脆的方法称之为明煅法。明煅法可使药物质地变得酥脆，其可能的原因包括：①煅烧使硫、砷、结晶水等物质挥发，以及氧化分解等反应，导致药物的分子结构发生变化，进而使药物的质地改变；②药物受热后不同组分在不同方向有着不同程度的胀缩，使药物晶格间产生了孔隙，质地变得酥脆。

煅淬法适用于质地坚硬，经过高温煅制仍不能酥脆的矿物药，以及临床上因特殊需要而必须煅淬的药物。自然铜经火煅后质地松脆易碎，二硫化铁分解成硫化铁，经醋淬后表面部分生成醋酸铁，使药物中铁离子溶出量增加，可增强散瘀止痛的作用。炉甘石经煅淬水飞后，质地纯洁细腻，适宜于眼科及外敷用，消除了由于颗粒较粗而造成的对局部黏膜的刺激性。

扣锅煅法适用于煅制质地疏松，炒炭易灰化和较难成炭的药物以及某些中成药在制备过程中需要综合制炭的药物。灯心草长于利水通淋，用于心烦失眠，尿少涩痛，口舌生疮；灯心草煅炭后可凉血止血，清热敛疮，外用治咽痹、乳蛾、阴疳。丝瓜络具有通络、活血、祛风、下乳的功效，生品长于祛风化痰，通络除痹；煅炭后有止血作用。

实验器材 •••

1. **仪器** 马弗炉，煅药炉，煅药锅，坩埚，坩埚钳，烧杯，量筒，电炉，乳钵，蒸发皿，搪瓷盘，台秤等。

2. **药材及试剂** 白矾，自然铜，炉甘石，灯心草，丝瓜络，米醋，河沙。

实验内容 •••

1. **明煅白矾** 取净白矾，置于煅锅内，用武火加热至融化，继续煅至膨胀松泡呈白色蜂窝状固体，完全干燥，停火，摊晾后取出，研成细粉。

2. **煅淬自然铜** 取净自然铜，置耐火容器内，用武火加热，煅至红透，取出，立即倒入醋液中浸淬。如此反复煅淬数次，至黑褐色，表面光泽消失并酥松，取出，放凉。每100kg自然铜，用米醋30kg。

3. **煅淬炉甘石** 取净炉甘石，置耐火容器内，用武火加热，煅至红透，取出，立即倒入水中浸淬，搅拌，倾取混悬液，残渣反复煅淬2至3次，合并混悬液，静置，倾去上层清水，取下层沉淀干燥，研细。

4. 灯心草炭 微课　　取净灯心草，扎成小把，置铁锅内，上扣一口径较小的锅，合缝处用河沙封固，在扣锅上压以重物，并贴一白纸或放数粒大米，用武火加热，煅至纸条或大米呈深黄色时停火，放冷后开锅取出。

5. 丝瓜络炭　　取净丝瓜络块，置铁锅内，上扣一口径较小的锅，合缝处用河沙封固，在扣锅上压以重物，并贴一白纸或放数粒大米，用武火加热，煅至纸条或大米呈深黄色时停火，放冷后开锅取出。

实验指导

1. 基本操作和操作注意点

（1）不同体积的药物要分开煅制。

（2）煅制过程不能停火。

（3）明煅法炮制药物时不能搅拌药物。

（4）自然铜煅制过程中会产生硫的升华物或有毒的二氧化硫气体，故应在通风处操作。

（5）闷煅时由于药物受热炭化，有大量气体及浓烟从锅缝中喷出，应随时堵封，以防空气进入使药物灰化。煅锅内药料不宜放得过多、过紧，以免煅制不透，影响质量。煅透后应放冷再开锅，以免药物遇空气后燃烧。

2. 实验报告格式

（1）实验目的

（2）实验原理

（3）实验内容

（4）讨论

3. 实验后思考

（1）明煅法炮制药物的目的是什么？

（2）煅淬法适用于哪类药物？

（3）煅炭和炒炭有哪些异同？

（郭常润　李兴华　陈玉江）

书网融合……

微课

Experiment 12 Representative Medicinal Processing of Calcining

◆ Experimental purposes

1. To master the methods of calcination, basic requirements.

2. To master the classification of calcination.

3. To understand the purpose of calcination.

◆ Experimental principle

The method of preparing drugs by calcination at high temperature is called calcination. According to the nature of the drug and calcination methods and requirements, it is divided into calcining openly, calcination and quenching, and the carbonizing by calcining (calcining above lidding a pot) .

The drug is placed directly in the smokeless furnace or refractory container calcination (not isolated air), so that the method of making drugs crisp is called calcining openly. Calcination method can make the drug texture brittle, the possible reasons include: calcination causes the drug in sulfur, arsenic, crystalline water and other substances volatile, or oxidation decomposition and other reactions, resulting in changes in the molecular structure of the drug, and then its texture changes; different components of the drug heated in different directions have different degrees of expansion and contraction, creating a gap between the drug lattice and making its texture brittle.

The calcining and quenching method is applicable to mineral drug with hard texture that cannot be crispy after high-temperature calcination, as well as drugs that must be calcined due to special clinical needs. After calcination, Pyritum has a brittle texture, and iron disulfide decomposes into iron sulfide. After being quenched with vinegar, the surface part generates iron acetate, which increases the amount of iron ions dissolved in the medicine and enhances the effect of dispersing blood stasis and relieving pain. After being calcined and quenched with water, Calamina has a pure and delicate texture, making it suitable for ophthalmology and external application, eliminating the irritation to local mucosa caused by its coarse particles.

The carbonizing by calcining method is suitable for calcining medicines with loose texture, which are easy to ash and difficult to carbonize when carbonizing, as well as some traditional Chinese patent medicines and simple preparations that need comprehensive carbonization during the preparation process. Junci Medulla is good at promoting diuresis, used for restlessness, insomnia, painful urination, and sores in the mouth and tongue; After calcining charcoal, it can cool blood and stop bleeding, clear heat and restrain sores, and be used externally to treat pharyngitis, breast moths, and Yin chancre. Loofah has the effects of clearing collaterals, promoting blood circulation, dispelling wind, and promoting milk. Raw products are better at dispelling weathered phlegm, clearing collaterals, and removing obstruction; Calcined charcoal has a hemostatic effect.

◆ Experimental apparatus

1. Instruments

Muffle furnace, drugs calcined furnace, calcined pan, crucible, crucible tongs, beaker, measuring cylinder, electric heater, mortar, evaporating dish, enamel tray, platform scale, et al.

2. Medicinal materials and chemicals

Alumen, Pyritum, Calamina, Junci Medulla, loofah, Vinegar, river sand.

◆ Experimental content

1. Calcining Alumen openly

Put the net alum in the calcining pot, and heat it with the fire until it melts; continue calcining until it swells and loosens the bubble and becomes white honeycomb solid; dry completely; cease fire; take it out after spreading and drying, and grind it into fine powder.

2. Calcining and quenching Pyritum

Take the clean drugs, put then in a refractory container and heat it on a strong fire, calcine crude drugs to red and immediately dip into vinegar quenching system, repeat this process 2-3 times until they are crisp enough, take the drugs out and cool. Use 30kg of vinegar per 100kg of Pyritum.

3. Calcining and quenching Calamina

Take the clean drugs, put them in a refractory container and heat it on a strong fire, calcine crude drugs to red and immediately dip into water quenching system, stirring and pouring suspension, repeat this process 2-3 times. Combine the suspension, stewing, pour the upper water and take the precipitate out, dry and grind into a powder.

4. Junci Medulla carbon

Take the clean Junci Medulla, bundle into small handfuls, and put it in a suitable container and attach a small one. Seal the joint of the two containers with river sand, put heavy weights on the smaller one, then paste a piece of white paper or put a few grains of rice, use a strong fire until white paper or rice becomes dark yellow, turn off the fire, allow to cool and take the medicines out.

5. Loofah carbon

Take the clean loofah, put it in a suitable container, attach a small one, seal their joint of with river sand, put heavy weights on the smaller container, paste a piece of white paper or put a few grains of rice, use a strong fire until the paper or rice becomes dark yellow, turn off the fire, allow to cool and take the medicines out.

◆ Experiment instruction

1. Primary operation and the notes of the operation

1.1 Different volumes of drugs to be calcined separately.

1.2 Calcination process cannot be ceased.

1.3 The drugs cannot be stirred in the calcination process.

1.4 The work should be done in a ventilated place as the calcining process of Pyritum will produce sulfur sublimates or toxic sulfur dioxide gases.

1.5 The work should be done in a suitable container, attach a small container, seal the joint of the two containers with river sand, allow to cool, and take the drugs out. But should be not put too more and too tight, 2/3 of the container is suitable.

2. Format of the experimental report

2.1 Purposes

2.2 Principle

2.3 The content of the experiment

2.4 Discussion

3. Considerations after the experiment

3.1 What is the purpose of the calcining openly?

3.2 Which kind of drug is suitable of calcining and quenching, carbonizing by calcining respectively?

3.3 What are the similarities and differences of calcining and quenching, carbonizing by calcining ?

(Edited by Changrun Guo, Xinghua Li and Yujiang Chen)

实验十三　自然铜及其炮制品中 Fe^{2+} 煎出量的测定

实验目的 •••

通过对自然铜炮制前后 Fe^{2+} 煎出量的比较，了解炮制自然铜的作用和意义。

实验原理 •••

自然铜为硫化物类矿物黄铁矿，其主要成分为二硫化铁（FeS_2）。据实验分析，铁约占46%，硫约占53%，并含有微量的铜、镍、锑、砷等。但由于产地不同，自然铜各组分含量也不同。

自然铜具有散瘀止痛，续筋接骨之效。生自然铜"燥性烈，易损人正气"，所以自然铜均需煅淬后应用，煅后自然铜质地酥脆，易于粉碎，水煎液中有效成分的煎出量增加，可增强其疗效。现代研究普遍认为，其中起主要治疗作用的是 Fe^{2+}，Fe^{2+} 具有促进骨髓生长、增加创口愈合强度和加强抗牵引力的作用。自然铜对实验性骨折具有促进愈合及增加愈合强度的作用。自然铜中的微量元素如 Hg、Cu、Ni、Sb 等也起协同作用。当水煎液中 Fe^{2+} 的含量增高时，其他元素的含量也增高；Fe^{2+} 含量降低时，其他元素含量也降低。Fe^{2+} 的测定方法多简便易行，干扰小，故可将 Fe^{2+} 的煎出量作为自然铜炮制的质量控制指标之一。

炮制的原理：在煅淬自然铜的过程中，会有下列反应发生：

$$(FeS_2)_2 \xrightarrow[\triangle]{400\,^\circ C} 2FeS + S_2$$

$$4FeS + 7O_2 \xrightarrow[\triangle]{500\,^\circ C} 2Fe_2S_3 + 4SO_2 \uparrow$$

$$6Fe_2O_3 \xrightarrow[\triangle]{>500\,^\circ C} 4Fe_3S_4 + O_2 \uparrow$$

实验器材 •••

1. 仪器　称量瓶，锥形瓶，量筒，漏斗，滤纸，酸式滴定管，电炉，玻棒等。

2. 药材及试剂　自然铜，活性炭，磷酸–硫酸混合液，二苯胺磺酸钠指示剂，0.025mol/L重铬酸钾标准液。

实验内容 •••

Fe^{2+} **煎出量的测定**　精密称取生、煅自然铜粉末各2g，置于250mL烧杯中，加水100mL，保持微沸25分钟，加入活性炭0.3g，继续煮沸5分钟，滤过，滤渣加80mL水，保持微沸20分钟，滤过，合并滤液（约50mL），放冷（或冷水降温）至室温。加入硫酸–磷酸混合液20mL，0.8%的二苯胺磺酸钠指示剂5滴，用0.025mol/L重铬酸钾标准液滴定至紫红色，按下式计算其百分含量：

$$6Fe^{2+} + Cr_2O_7^{2-} \rightleftharpoons 6Fe^{3+} + 2Cr^{3+} + 3H_2O$$

$$Fe^{2+}\% = \frac{N_{K_2Cr_2O_7} V_{K_2Cr_2O_7} \times 55.85/1000}{W} \times 100\%$$

实验指导 •••

1. 预习

（1）自然铜在煅制后外观发生什么变化？成分发生什么变化？

（2）自然铜中对人体有害的元素经过炮制后有什么量与质的改变？

（3）测定Fe^{2+}时，所选用的指示剂二苯胺磺酸钠的终点变色有什么条件要求？和实验中所加的混酸有无关系？

2. 基本操作和操作注意点

（1）基本操作　①掌握自然铜水煎液中Fe^{2+}的测定方法；②正确进行滴定操作。

（2）操作注意点　① 在煅制自然铜的过程中，会产生硫的升华物或有毒的二氧化硫气体，故操作应在通风橱内进行，且要注意劳动保护。② 醋淬时自然铜要趁热投入醋中，且应迅速捞出，不可在醋液中久泡。③ 除可在马弗炉中进行煅制外，还可用煤油炉或煤球炉等。由于它们散热快，温度可相应提高，可用热电偶或测电笔测定煅药铁锅内的温度，以不超过500℃为宜。④ 在电炉上煎煮时，电压不宜高，避免煎液向外迸溅，且需经常搅拌，防止在瓶底结块；加活性炭时需离火，以免引起爆沸。⑤ 滤液需冷至室温后方可滴定，否则对含量测定有影响。⑥ 滴定时间不宜长，否则结果偏大。

3. 实验报告格式

（1）实验目的

（2）实验原理

（3）实验内容及计算结果

Fe^{2+}煎出量的测定

表 13-1　自然铜煅制前后Fe^{2+}的百分含量

样品	重量（g）	消耗的重铬酸钾溶液（mL）	百分含量（%）
自然铜			
煅自燃铜			

（4）讨论

4. 实验后思考

（1）中医为何多用煅自然铜？

（2）用重铬酸钾法测定Fe^{2+}含量时，滴定前为什么要加入硫酸-磷酸混合酸？加入该混合酸后为何要立即滴定？另外，你还可以举出哪几种测定Fe^{2+}含量的方法？

（3）你认为在煅制矿物药的研究中，除主要成分的含量测定外，还可以进行哪些方面的研究？

（郭常润　陈玉江）

Experiment 13   The Assay of the Fe^{2+} Content of the Crude and the Processed Pyritum in the Water - soluble Extractives

◆ Experimental purpose

To understand the calcining meanings of the Pyritum by assaying the ferrocyanide ion content before and after processing.

◆ Experimental principle

Pyritum is a mineral of sulfide of Pyrite group, mainly containing sulfide. By analysis, it contains 46% iron and 53% sulfide approximately with some trace compounds such as copper, nickel, arsenic, antimony, and cobalt. Due to the difference of the producing sites, the content of each compound in Pyritum is different.

Pyritum can eliminate blood stasis, relieve pain and reunite fractured bones and restorate injured muscles and tendons. The crude Pyritum has strong dryness and easily violates the human bodies genuine energy, so it must be tempered before used. After being calcined, Pyritum becomes crisp and easy to be powdered. The efficient ingredients content can increase in the water-soluble extractives and the curative effect can be strengthened. Researches generally confirm that the major efficient ingredient is ferrocyanide ion contained in Pyritum. Ferrocyanide ion is able to accelerate the growth of bone marrow, enhance the strength of the recovery from wound and increase the intensity of anti-traction. It is reported that the Pyritum can accelerate the recovery and improve the strength of the experimental broken bone. Hence, we can conclude that the effects of ferrocyanide ion and Pyritum are in agreement. The trace compounds in Pyritum such as mercury, copper, nickel and antimony have symergistic actions. Experiments show that the other compounds contents in the water-soluble extractives will be increased when ferro-cyanide ion content increased. The methods of assaying ferrocyanide ion content are handy and not so easy to be interfered, so we regard the ferrocyanide ion content as the criterion to control the quality of Pyritum.

The principle of processing: when processing Pyritum, the following reactions will take place:

$$(FeS_2)_2 = \frac{400\,℃}{\triangle} 2FeS + S_2$$

$$4FeS + 7O_2 = \frac{500\,℃}{\triangle} 2Fe_2S_3 + 4SO_2 \uparrow$$

$$6Fe_2O_3 = \frac{>500\,℃}{\triangle} 4Fe_3S_4 + O_2 \uparrow$$

We use potassium dichromate titration in Oxidation-reduction titration to assay the ferrocyanide ion content in Pyritum.

◆ Experimental apparatus

1. Instruments

Triangular beaker, measuring cylinder, funnel, filter paper, acid buret, electric furnace, transformer, et al.

2. Medicinal materials and chemicals

Pyritum, activated carbon, the mixed acid of sulfuric acid and phosphoric acid, indicator of sodium diphenylamine sulfonate, 0.025mol/L potassium dichromate TS.

◆ Experimental content

Assay of ferrocyanide ion content

Weigh accurately 2g Pyritum and calcined Pyritum into 250mL triangular beakers, respectively. Add 100mL water and boil for 25 minutes. Add activated carbon, continue to boil for 5 min and filter. Add 80mL water to the residue, then boil for 20 minutes and filter. Mix the two filtrates (50mL) and cool in air or in the cold water at room temperature. Add 20mL mixed acid and 5 drops of 10% sodium diphenylamine sulfonate and titrate with 0.025mol/L potassium dichromate until the color of the solution turns purplish-red. Assay the ferrocyanide ion content according to the following formula:

$$6Fe^{2+} + Cr_2O_7^{2-} \rightleftharpoons 6Fe^{3+} + 2Cr^{3+} + 3H_2O$$

$$Fe^{2+}\% = \frac{N_{K_2Cr_4O_7} V_{K_2Cr_4O_7} \times 55.85/1000}{W} \times 100\%$$

◆ Experimental instruction

1. Preview

1.1 What changes take place in the appearance of Pyritum after calcining? How about its efficient ingredients?

1.2 What quantitative and qualitative changes of the compounds poisonous for human bodies in Pyritum take place after calcining?

1.3 In the process of assaying the ferrocyanide ion content, what conditions are needed for sodium diphenylamine sulfonate as indicator? Is there any relationship to the mixed acid?

2. Primary operations and notes of the operations

2.1 Primary operations

2.1.1 Master the assaying methods of the ferrocyanide ion content in the water-soluble extractives of Pyritum.

2.1.2 Conducting correct titrating operation.

2.2 Notes of the operations

2.2.1 The sublimation of sulfur or poisonous gas or sulfur dioxide would be produced in the process of calcining Pyritum. Therefore, the operations should be carried out in the ventilated room and the operators are needed to be protected.

2.2.2 When tempered with vinegar, Pyritum must be put into the vinegar when hot, and should be taken out quickly and cannot be soaked in it for a long time.

2.2.3 We may use kerosene furnace or egg-shaped briquet furnace in addition to muffle furnace because they scatter heat quickly and can increase the temperature. We may measure the temperature with thermocouple or test pencil. The optimum temperature is 500℃.

2.2.4 When boiling on the electric furnace, the voltage should not be very high in order to avoid the spillage of solution. Meanwhile, it should be agitated continuously to avoid the gathering into solid. The activated carbon should be put away from fire when added to avoid boiling violently.

2.2.5 Titration operation con not be conducted until the filtrate is cooled to room temperature. Otherwise, it will influence the assay of the content.

2.2.6 The time used to titrate should not be too long. Otherwise, the results will become bigger.

3. Format of the experimental report

3.1 Object

3.2 Principle

3.3 Experimental data and calculational results

Table 13-1   Content of Pyritum and Pyritum calcined

Sample	Weight (g)	The volume of solution of potassium dichromate used (mL)	Content (%)
Pyritum			
Pyritum calcined			

3.4 Discussion

4. Considerations after the experiment

4.1 Why do TCM doctors use mostly calcined Pyritum?

4.2 Why adding the mixed acid before titration when measuring the ferrocyanide ion content using potassium dichromate titration? Why titrating promptly as soon as adding the mixed acid? In addition, what methods can you think of to measure the ferrocyanide ion content?

4.3 In your opinion, which researches should also be carried out to investigate the calcined mineral medicines, in addition to assaying the primary ingredients content?

(Edited by Changrun Guo and Yujiang Chen)

第五章 蒸 法

实验十四 蒸法的代表药物炮制

实验目的 •••

1. 掌握制何首乌的炮制方法、注意事项及成品质量评价标准。
2. 熟悉何首乌炮制的目的和意义。

实验原理 •••

何首乌生品具有解毒、消痈、截疟、润肠通便的功效，可用于疮痈、瘰疬、风疹瘙痒、久疟体虚、肠燥便秘等。经黑豆汁拌蒸后，味转甘厚而性转温，增强了补肝肾、益精血、乌须发、强筋骨、化浊降脂的作用；并消除了滑肠致泻的不良反应。

实验器材 •••

1. **仪器** 蒸锅，蒸笼，电子秤，烧杯，搪瓷盘等。
2. **药材** 何首乌，黑豆。

实验内容 •••

1. **制何首乌** 取何首乌片或块，置非铁质的适宜容器内，照蒸法清蒸或用黑豆汁拌匀后蒸，蒸至内外均呈棕褐色，或晒至半干，切片，干燥。每100kg何首乌片（块），用黑豆10kg。
2. **黑豆汁制法** 取黑豆10kg，加水适量，煮约4小时，熬汁约15kg，豆渣再加水煮约3小时，熬汁约10kg，合并得黑豆汁约25kg。

实验指导 •••

1. **基本操作和操作注意点**
（1）应待黑豆汁被何首乌吸尽后再蒸制。
（2）蒸制时要注意火候，若时间太短则达不到目的；若蒸过久，则影响药效，并且致使水分过高，难以干燥。

2. **实验报告格式**
（1）实验目的
（2）实验原理
（3）实验内容
（4）讨论

3. **实验后思考**
古人对于何首乌的炮制用具提出了"忌铁"的要求，原因是什么？

（李兴华　陈玉江）

Experiment 14   Representative Medicinal Processing of Steaming Method

◆ Experimental purposes

1. To master the basic operations, precautions, and quality evaluation standards of steaming Polygoni Multiflori Radix.

2. To familiarize the purpose and significance of steaming Polygoni Multiflori Radix.

◆ Experimental principle

The crude drug of Polygoni Multiflori Radix can counteract toxicity, cure carbuncles and relax bowels. Thus, it is used in the treatments for constipation, carbuncles, hyperlipemia and tuberculosis of lymphatic glands et al. Mixed with black bean juice after steaming, Polygoni Multiflori Radix Praeparata can be used to invigorate the liver and the kidney, replenish vital essence and blood, blacken the hair, and strengthen the tendon and bones. It can also be used to treat hyperlipemia, and eliminate the side effects of diarrhea caused by slippery intestines.

◆ Experimental apparatus

1. Instruments

Stainless steel pot, food steamer, counter balance, beaker, enamel tray, et al

2. Medicinal materials

Polygoni Multiflori Radix, black bean.

◆ Experimental content

1. Polygoni Multiflori Radix praeparata

Slices or pieces of Polygoni Multiflori Radix are mixed with black bean juice. According to method, strewing is carried out in a suitable non-ferrous container until the juice is exhausted or its pieces is steamed alone or after being mixed with black bean juice to a brown color, or dried under the sun to partial dryness, and then cut into slices and dried.

For each 100kg of slices or pieces of Polygoni Multiflori Radix, 10kg of black beans is used.

2. Preparation of black bean juice

10kg of black beans in an appropriate amount of water is boiled for about 4 hours and stewed to obtain about 15kg of black bean juice. The bean residue is boiled again in water for about 3 hours and stewed to obtain about 10kg of juice and combined to obtain about 25kg of the black bean juice.

◆ Experiment instruction

1. Primary operation and the notes of the operation

1.1 It should be steamed after the black bean juice is sucked up by Polygoni Multiflori Radix.

1.2 When steaming, attention should be paid to the heat. If the time is too short, the purpose cannot be achieved; If steamed too long, it will affect the efficacy and cause excessive moisture, making it difficult to dry.

2. Format of the experimental report

2.1 Purposes

2.2 Principle

2.3 The content of the experiment

2.4 Discussion

3. Considerations after the experiment

What is the reason of ancient people put forward the requirement of "avoiding iron" for the processing of Polygoni Multiflori Radix ?

（Edited by Xinghua Li and Yujiang Chen）

实验十五 黄芩及其炮制品中黄芩苷的含量测定

实验目的 ●●●

1. 掌握用HPLC法测定黄芩及其不同炮制品中黄芩苷的含量。

2. 通过比较黄芩在炮制前后黄芩苷的含量变化，了解炮制对黄芩的作用和意义。

3. 通过比较用不同的软化方法获得各种黄芩中黄芩苷的含量，确定软化的最佳方式。

实验原理 ●●●

黄芩为唇形科植物黄芩 *Scutellaria baicalensis* Georgi. 的干燥根。本品苦、寒，可清热燥湿，泻火解毒，止血安胎。用于湿温、暑温、呕恶，湿热痞满，泻痢黄疸，肺热咳嗽，高热烦渴，胎动不安等症。黄芩沸水煮或蒸制，使药材软化，便于切片。生黄芩性苦，微寒，以清热泻火力强，多用于风热湿症。酒制入血分，并可借助酒的升腾之力，治疗目赤肿痛，上焦肺热及四肢肌表之湿热；同时，因酒大热，可缓和黄芩苦寒之性，以免伤及脾胃，导致腹痛。黄芩炒后可去寒性以清热燥湿，和胃安胎力胜，多用于痢疾、湿温和胎动不安。

现代研究认为，黄芩遇冷水变绿，是由于黄芩中所含的酶在一定的温度和湿度条件下，可酶解其中的黄芩苷，使之变成黄芩苷元和汉黄芩素。其中的黄芩苷元本身不稳定，易被氧化变绿。黄芩苷的水解与酶的活性有关，以冷水浸时酶的活性最大，而经蒸、煮、炒以后就可以破坏酶，使其失活，从而达到杀酶保苷的目的。

实验器材 ●●●

1. 仪器 索式提取器，1000mL容量瓶2只，细筛（60目），高效液相色谱仪，滤纸，脱脂棉。

2. 药材及试剂 黄芩（药材），黄芩苷对照品（中国食品药品检定研究院提供），乙腈，无水乙醇，蒸馏水，磷酸，甲醇。

实验内容 ●●●

黄芩苷的含量测定

（1）色谱条件与系统适用性试验 用十八烷基硅烷键合硅胶为填充剂；色谱柱为C_{18}柱，柱温为35℃，流动相为乙腈–0.6%磷酸水溶液（21∶79），检测波长为274nm。按黄芩苷峰计算，理论塔板数应不低于2500。

（2）对照品溶液的制备 精密称取60℃减压干燥4小时的黄芩苷对照品适量，加甲醇制成每1mL含60μg黄芩苷的溶液即得。

（3）供试品溶液的制备 分别精密称取黄芩生品及炮制品细粉（60目）0.3 g，置于100mL量瓶中，加70%的乙醇至刻度，摇匀，称定重量，超声提取30分钟，取出，室温下冷却1小时，用70%乙醇补足减失重量，摇匀，滤过，取续滤液1mL置10mL量瓶中，加甲醇稀释至刻度，摇匀。

（4）标准曲线的制备 分别精密吸取上述对照品液1mL、2mL、3mL、4mL、5mL、6mL，分别以甲醇定容至10mL，分别精取10μL，注入色谱柱进行测定。以峰面积为纵坐标，样品浓度（μg/mL）为横坐标，绘制标准曲线，得回归方程。

（5）样品含量测定 分别精密吸取对照品几种样品液各10μL进样，求得各样品峰面积，代入回归方程计算样品的含量。

实验指导 •••

1.预习 黄芩苷的含量测定方法有哪些?

2.基本操作和操作注意点

(1)基本操作 掌握黄芩苷的含量测定方法。

(2)操作注意点 黄芩苷进行含量测定时要注意流动相中水的比例和柱温的变化。

3.实验报告格式

(1)实验目的

(2)实验原理

(3)实验内容及计算结果

黄芩苷的含量测定

表 15-1 黄芩苷的含量测定

样品	重量(g)	峰面积	样品浓度(μg/mL)	百分含量(%)
冷浸黄芩片				
蒸黄芩片				
煮黄芩片				
酒黄芩				
黄芩炭				

(4)讨论

4.思考题

(1)黄芩苷为何不稳定?在加工软化和炮制时要注意哪些问题?

(2)影响黄芩饮片质量的因素有几种?是如何影响的?你可以设计一套黄芩软化切片和炮制的方案吗?

(季 德 陈玉江)

Experiment 15　The Assay of the Baicalin in the Crude and the Processed Scutellariae Radix

◆ Experimental purposes

1. To master the HPLC method of determining the content of baicalin in different processed drugs.

2. To study the principle and significance of processing through the comparison of the baicalin content after and before processing.

3. To determine the optimum method of softening by comparing the baicalin content using different softening method.

◆ Experimental principle

Scutellariae Radix is the dried root of *Scutellaria baicalensis* Georgi (Fam. Labiatae). The attributes of prepared Scutellariae Radix are bitter in taste, and cold in nature. The drug can remove damp-heat, quench fire, counteract toxicity and arrest bleeding, safeguard foetus. It can be used in many indications such as test, nausea and vomiting in epidemic febrile diseases caused by damp-heat or summer-heat; feeling stuffiness in the abdomen, acute dysentery or jaundice caused by damp-heat; cough due to heat in the lung; high fever with fire thirst; spitting of blood and epistaxis due to heat in blood; carbuncles and sores; threatened abortion. The method of boiling and braising can make the drug soft, which is convenient for slicing. The crude drug is good at removing damp-heat, quench fire, and usually used in febrile diseases caused by damp-heat or summer-heat. Wine into the blood, and aided by the ascending power of alcohol, which is especially good for the diseases of eye sore, heat in lung and the damp-heat in limb and skin. At the same time, with the heat property of wine, the cold property of drug is decreased, so as to avoid injuring the spleen and stomach, resulting in abdominal pain. The function of removing damp-heat, quenching fire will be strengthened after the stir-frying, and it also could be used in dysentery, damp-heat and fetal irritability.

Modern studies show that the reason why Scutellariae Radix turns green when it is exposed to cold water is that the enzyme contained in Scutellariae Radix can enzymatically hydrolyze baicalin under certain temperature and humidity conditions to make it become baicalin and wogonin. Because baicalin is unstable, it is easy to be oxidized and turn green. The drug will lose a lot of baicalin when it is soaked in cold water due to the highest activity of the enzyme, while the drug processed through boiling, steaming and stir-frying can reserve the most of baicalin because the heat processing can destroy the enzyme to protect the baicalin.

◆ Instruments and chemicals

1. Instruments

Extractor, two 1000mL volumetric flasks, fine sieve (NO.60 sieve), HPLC, filter paper, absorbent cotton.

2. Medicinal materials and chemicals

Scutellariae Radix, wine, baicalin (provided by National Institutes for Food and Drug Control), Acetonitrile (AR), alcohol (AR), distilled water, phosphoric acid (AR), Methanol (AR).

◆ Experimental content

Assay of effective compound

1.1 Chromatographic system and system suitability

Use octadecylsilane bonded silica gel as the stationary phase, column temperature is 35℃ and acetonitrile-0.6% phosphoric acid（21：79）as the mobile phase. The wavelength of the detector is 274nm. The number of theoretical plates of the column is not less than 2500, calculated with the reference to the peak of baicalin.

1.2 Preparation of reference solution

Weigh accurately a quantity of baicalin CRS, dried in vacuum at 60℃ for 4 hours, dissolve in methanol to produce a solution containing 60μg per 1mL as the reference solution.

1.3 Preparation of test solution

Weigh accurately 0.3g powder（60 mesh）into a 100mL volumetric flask, add 70% alcohol to the scale, shake and mix well, weigh accurately and extract for 30 minutes under ultrasonic, take out, cool at room temperature for 1 hour, dilute with 70% alcohol to the scale, shake well, and filter. Transfer 1mL successive filtrate to the 10mL volumetric, dilute with methanol to the scale and mix well.

1.4 Preparation of calibration curve

Transfer accurately 1, 2, 3, 4, 5, 6mL reference solution to 10mL volumetric flasks, dissolve and dilute with methanol to the scale, respectively. Accurately inject 10μL each reference solution, respectively, into the column. With the peak area as the y-axis, the content of the sample as the x-axis, draw the calibration curve to get the regression equation.

1.5 Measurement of the sample content

Inject accurately 10μL sample solutions respectively to the column, get the peak area, and take it into the regression equation to obtain the sample content.

◆ Experimental instruction

1. Preview

What methods could be used to determine the content of baicalin?

2. Primary operations and notes of the operations

2.1 Primary operations

Master the determining method of baicalin with HPLC.

2.2 Notes of the operations

When determining the content of baicalin, attention should be paid to the change of water ratio in mobile phase and column temperature.

3. Format of the experimental report

3.1 Object

3.2 Principle

3.3 Content and calculating results

Determining the content of baicalin

Table 15-1 Assay of baicalin

Sample	Weight (g)	Peak area	Sample content (μg/mL)	Percentages (%)
Drug rinsed in cold water				
Drug steamed in hot water				
Drug boiled in hot water				
Drug stir-frying with wine				
Drug carbonizing				

3.4 Discussion

4. Considerations after the experiment

4.1 Why is the baicalin not stable? What problem should you note when soften and process the drug?

4.2 How many factors can affect the quality of Scutellariae Radix slices? How do they affect it? Can you design a scheme to soften and process it?

（ Edited by De Ji and Yujiang Chen ）

实验十六　何首乌及其炮制品中成分含量分析

实验目的 ●●●

通过对何首乌炮制前后各成分的含量测定，了解何首乌炮制以后功效改变及泻下作用减弱的原理。

实验原理 ●●●

何首乌为蓼科植物何首乌 *Polygonum multiflorum* Thunb. 的块根。生首乌能解毒，散结，滑肠致泻。炮制后味变甘苦，性温，功效长于补肝肾，益精血，所以其制品为常用滋补药之一。

何首乌的成分主要是羟基蒽醌衍生物、卵磷脂和芪类化合物，其中结合蒽醌具有泻下作用。何首乌经过炮制，使部分结合蒽醌衍生物水解为无致泻作用的游离蒽醌衍生物，从而大大地减弱了泻下作用，而何首乌中其他有效成分，如芪类化合物，其含量略有升高，所以炮制后，何首乌不仅消除了其泻下作用，还增强了滋补作用。

本实验应用比色法测定何首乌炮制后游离蒽醌及结合蒽醌的含量变化，采用一阶导数光谱法测定芪类化合物含量。

实验器材 ●●●

1. 仪器　紫外可见分光光度计，高效液相色谱仪，烧杯（500mL），容量瓶（10mL、25mL、50mL），移液管（0.5mL、1mL、2mL、5mL），量筒（50mL、100mL），称量瓶，索氏提取器，溶剂回收装置，吸管，圆底烧瓶（50mL、100mL），漏斗，分液漏斗，锥形瓶（250mL），滤纸，玻棒，脱脂棉。

2. 药材及试剂　0.5%醋酸镁甲醇溶液，三氯甲烷（AR），2.5 mol/L硫酸，无水硫酸钠，大黄素标准品，2，3，5，4'–四羟基芪–2-*O*-*β*-D-葡萄糖苷标准品，生、制首乌。

实验内容 ●●●

1. 炮制前后何首乌中蒽醌类成分的测定

（1）标准曲线的制备　精密称取5.0mg大黄素置50mL容量瓶中，加乙醚溶解稀释至刻度，配制成浓度为0.1mg/mL的标准溶液。精密吸取1.00mL、2.00mL、3.00mL、4.00mL、5.00mL上述溶液，分别置于25mL容量瓶中，在40℃水浴上蒸去乙醚，残渣用0.5%醋酸镁甲醇溶液溶解并稀释至刻度，摇匀，于513 nm处测定吸收度，以0.5%醋酸镁甲醇溶液作空白对照，绘制吸收度–浓度曲线。

（2）何首乌中游离蒽醌的测定　精密称取生首乌、制首乌0.4g，分别置于30mL索氏提取器中，加三氯甲烷30mL回流提取至无色（约1小时），回收三氯甲烷至干，残渣加少量0.5%醋酸镁甲醇溶液溶解，转移至25mL容量瓶中，并稀释至刻度，摇匀，于513nm处测定吸收度，以0.5%醋酸镁甲醇溶液作空白对照，由标准曲线查得浓度，并计算其百分含量。

（3）何首乌中结合蒽醌的含量测定　精密称取生首乌、制首乌粉末（过60目筛）各0.2g，分别置于100mL圆底烧瓶中，加2.5mol/L硫酸30mL，直火水解1小时，冷却后加入三氯甲烷30mL，水浴回流12分钟，冷却后，以脱脂棉过滤至分液漏斗中，分取三氯甲烷层，酸水液置100mL圆底烧瓶中，再加三氯甲烷30mL，继续回流15分钟，冷却，过滤，分取三氯甲烷层，水层再用三氯甲烷萃取2次，每次10mL，合并三氯甲烷液，用少量蒸馏水洗至中性后，加无水硫酸钠脱水，过滤，回收三氯甲烷至干，按游离蒽醌测定法测定。利用标准曲线求得各样品液的浓度（mg/mL）计算得总蒽醌含量，由总蒽醌含量减去游离蒽醌含量即得结合蒽醌含量。

计算式：

$$含量\% = （C \times T） / （W \times 1000） \times 100\%$$

式中，C 为由标准曲线求得的样品的浓度（mg/mL）；T 为稀释度；W 为样品的重量（g）。

2. 炮制前后何首乌中茋类成分的含量测定

（1）标准曲线的绘制　精密称取 2,3,5,4'- 四羟基茋 -2-O-β-D- 葡萄糖苷 2.5mg，置 50mL 容量瓶中，用 95% 乙醇溶解稀释至刻度，摇匀，分别吸取此溶液 0.5mL、1.0mL、2.0mL、3.0mL、4.0mL、5.0mL 于 10mL 容量瓶中，加 95% 乙醇稀释至刻度，摇匀，则得浓度分别为 2.5μg/mL、5.0μg/mL、10.0 μg/mL、15.0μg/mL、20.0μg/mL、25.0μg/mL 的 2,3,5,4'- 四羟基茋 -2-O-β-D- 葡萄糖苷乙醇溶液，以乙醇作空白对照，在紫外可见分光光度计上测定各自溶液在 330nm、334nm 波长处的吸收值，以 $\triangle A$（$A_{334} - A_{330}$）对浓度作标准曲线。

（2）何首乌中茋类的含量测定　取生首乌、制首乌粉末（过 60 目筛）各 0.05g，分别置于圆底烧瓶中，加入 95% 乙醇 80mL 提取 2 小时后，将提取液转移至 100mL 容量瓶中，用 95% 乙醇溶解稀释至刻度，摇匀。以 95% 乙醇作空白，在 330nm、334nm 波长处测定 A_{334}、A_{330} 值，从标准曲线上求得生首乌和制首乌中茋类化合物的浓度 C（mg/mL），并计算出样品的百分含量。

$$百分含量 = （C \times T） / （W \times 1000） \times 100\%$$

式中，C 为由标准曲线求得的量（mg/mL）；T 为稀释度；W 为样品的重量（g）。

3. 炮制前后何首乌中 2,3,5,4'- 四羟基二苯乙烯 -2-O-β-D- 葡萄糖苷含量测定

色谱条件与系统适用性试验　以十八烷基硅烷键合硅胶为填充剂；以乙腈 - 水（25∶75）为流动相；检测波长为 320nm。理论板数按 2,3,5,4'- 四羟基二苯乙烯 -2-O-β-D- 葡萄糖苷峰计算应不低于 2000。

对照品溶液的制备　取 2,3,5,4'- 四羟基二苯乙烯 -2-O-β-D- 葡萄糖苷对照品适量，精密称定，加稀乙醇制成每 1mL 含 0.2mg 的溶液，即得。

供试品溶液的制备　各取何首乌和制首乌粉末（过四号筛）约 0.2g，精密称定，置具塞锥形瓶中，精密加入稀乙醇 25mL，称定重量，加热回流 30 分钟，放冷，再称定重量，用稀乙醇补足减失的重量，摇匀，静置，上清液滤过，取续滤液，即得。

测定法　分别精密吸取对照品溶液与供试品溶液各 10μL，注入液相色谱仪，测定，计算，即得。

实验指导 •••

1. 预习

（1）何首乌属于哪一科哪一属的药用植物？其功效、性味如何？经炮制后其功效、性味又有何变化？

（2）何首乌主要含有哪些有效成分？各成分有何作用？

（3）辅料黑豆的功效与首乌的功效之间有什么协同关系？

（4）复习一阶导数光谱法的使用原理。

2. 基本操作和操作注意点

（1）基本操作　①正确使用索氏提取器；②正确使用紫外可见分光光度计和高效液相色谱仪。

（2）操作注意点　①本实验使用有机溶剂，实验室内严禁明火；②制首乌需充分粉碎，否则将因生首乌易粉碎而造成生、制品粒度差别，会给实验结果带来较大误差；③使用三氯甲烷提取及回收溶剂时，应严格控制温度，温度过高，会在加入醋酸镁甲醇溶液比色时产生极大的颜色误差。

3. 实验报告格式

（1）实验目的

（2）实验原理

（3）实验内容及计算结果

表 16-1　何首乌及其炮制品中蒽醌成分含量测定结果

样品	样品重量（g）	A（游）	A（总）	游离蒽醌（%）	结合蒽醌（%）	总蒽醌（%）
生首乌						
制首乌						

表 16-2　何首乌及其炮制品中芪类含量测定结果

样品	样品重量（g）	A_{330}	A_{334}	ΔA	C（mg/mL）	含量（%）
生首乌						
制首乌						

表 16-3　何首乌炮制前后二苯乙烯苷的含量

样品	样品重量（g）	峰面积	浓度（μg/mL）	百分含量（%）
生首乌				
制首乌				

（4）讨论

4. 思考题

（1）何首乌的炮制方法有哪几种？炮制后，其泻下作用为何缓解？

（2）中药中蒽醌类、芪类的定量测定方法还有哪些？

（季　德　陈玉江）

Experiment 16　The Change of the Ingredient Contents in Polygoni Multiflori Radix after Processing

◆ Experimental purpose

To study the principle of the pharmacodynamics change and the attenuation of purging action through the assay of the crude and the processed drug.

◆ Experimental principle

Polygoni Multiflori Radix is the dried root tuber of *Polygonum Multiflorum* Thunb.（Fam. Polygonaceae）. The crude drug is used to counteract toxicity, cure carbuncles and relax bowels. The attributes of processed Polygoni Multiflori Radix are bitter in taste, and warm in nature. Its functions are superior to invigorate the liver and kidney and to replenish the vital essence and blood. So, the processed Polygoni Multiflori Radix is usually used as a nourishing drug.

The principal components of the drug are the derivant of hydroxyanthraquinone, lecithin and stilbenoids. The conjugated anthraquinone possesses the purging function. After processed, the conjugated anthraquinone will partly turn into free anthraquinone which has not such function, while the content of other ingredients such as stilbenoids, rises mildly. The processing not only eliminates the purging action but also enhances the nourishing action of the drug.

This experiment applies colorimetric method to determine the content of the free and conjugated anthraquinone of the crude and processed drug, adopts primary derivative spectrometry to determine the content of stilbenoids.

◆ Experimental apparatus

1. Instruments

Spectrophotometer, HPLC, beaker（500mL）, measuring flask（10, 25, 50mL）, pipette（0.5, 1, 2, 5mL）, measuring cylinder（50, 100mL）, weighing bottle, Soxhlet's extractor, solvent recovery apparatus, pipette, round bottom flask（50, 100mL）funnel, separating funnel, conical flask（250mL）, filter paper, glass rod, absorbent cotton.

2. Medicinal materials and chemicals

0.5%mgAc$_2$-MeOH, CHCl$_3$（AR）, 2.5 mol/L H$_2$SO$_4$, anhydrous sodium sulfate, emodin CRS, 2,3,5,4'-Tetrahydroxystilbene-2-*O*-*β*-D-glucoside standard, crude and processed, Polygoni Multiflori Radix pieces.

◆ Experimental content

1. Determine the anthraquinone of raw and processed Polygoni Multiflori Radix

1.1 Standard curve

Weigh accurately 5.0mg of emodin in a 50mL volumetric flask, dissolve in an appropriate quantity of ether and dilute to volume, mix well, as the reference solution（containing 0.1mg of emodin per 1mL）. Measure accurately 1.00, 2.00, 3.00, 4.00 and 5.00mL of the reference solution in 25mL volumetric flasks separately.

Evaporate the ether to dryness on a water bath at 40℃, dissolve the residue in an appropriate quantity of 0.5%MgAc$_2$-MeOH and dilute to volume, mix well. Measure the absorbance at 513nm, take the solution of 0.5%MgAc$_2$-MeOH as a blank, and plot the standard curve with absorbance as ordinate and concentration as abscissa.

1.2 Assay of the free anthraquinone of the drug

Weigh accurately 0.4g of the crude and processed Polygoni Multiflori Radix in two 30mL Soxhlet's extractors separately. Heat under reflux extraction with 30mL chloroform until the chloroform in the Soxhlet's extractors becomes colorless (about 1 hour). Recover the chloroform to dryness on a water bath and dissolve the residue in a small quantity of solution of 0.5%MgAc$_2$-MeOH. Divert equivalently the solution into a 25mL volumetric flask, dilute to scale with 0.5%MgAc$_2$-MeOH, mix well. Measure the absorbance at 513nm, take the solution of 0.5%MgAc$_2$-MeOH as the blank group, read out the concentration from the standard curve, and calculate its content.

1.3 Assay of the conjugated anthraquinone of the drug

Weigh accurately 0.2g of the power of crude and processed Polygoni Multiflori Radix (both through No.60 sieve) in two 100mL round bottom flasks separately. Add 30mL of 2.5mol/L sulfuric acid, hydrolyze for 1 hour on bare fire, let it cool, add 30mL chloroform, heat under reflux on a water bath for 15 minutes, cool it again. Filter the solution in a 125mL separating funnel with some absorbent cotton, separate the chloroform layer, transfer the acid liquor to a 100mL round bottom flask, add 30mL chloroform again, continue to heat under reflux on a water bath for 15 minutes, allow to cool and filter, separate the chloroform layer, extract the water layer with chloroform twice, 10mL each time, combine the chloroform extractions, wash them with a small quantity of distilled water to neutrality, dehydrate with anhydrous sodium sulfate, filter, recover the chloroform to dry, determine the content according to the method of the free anthraquinone. The concentration on the standard curve is used to calculate the total anthraquinone content, and the combined anthraquinone content is the total anthraquinone content minus the free anthraquinone content.

Formula:

$$Content(\%) = (C \times T)/(W \times 1000) \times 100\%$$

Note:

C: The amount obtained from the standard curve (mg/mL); T: The dilution; W: The weight of the sample (g).

2. Assay of the stilbenoids of the crude and processed drug

2.1 Standard curve: Weigh accurately 2.5mg of 2,3,5,4'-tetrahydroxystilbene-2-O-β-D-glucoside in a 50mL volumetric flask, dissolve in an appropriate quantity of 95% ethanol and dilute to volume, and shake well. Transfer accurately 0.5, 1.0, 2.0, 3.0, 4.0, 5.0mL of the solution to volumetric flasks separately, dilute to volume with 95% ethanol, and mix well. Then, the concentrations of polydatin are 2.5, 5.0, 10.0, 15.0, 20.0, 25.0μg/mL in the solutions respectively. Measure the absorbance by spectrophotometer at 330 nm and 334 nm, take the ethanol as the blank group, plot the standard curve, using $\triangle A$ (A_{334}–A_{330}) as ordinate and concentration as abscissa.

2.2 Assay: Weigh 0.05g the power of crude and processed drug (both through No.60 sieve) in two extractors separately, each add 80mL of 95% ethanol, heat under reflex for 2 hours until the stilbenoids are extracted thoroughly, divert all the extraction liquor into a 100mL volumetric flask, dilute with 95% ethanol to volume, and mix well.

Measure the absorbance at 330nm add 334nm, taking the ethanol as the blank group, calculate the percentage content from the regression equation or the standard curve.

Formula:

$$Content(\%)=(C \times T)/(W \times 1000) \times 100\%$$

Note:

C: The amount obtained from the standard curve(mg/mL); T: The dilution; W: The weight of the sample(g).

3. Assay of 2,3,5,4'-tetrahydroxystilbene-2-O-β-D-glucopyranoside

3.1 Chromatographic condition: Chromatographic column is C18. Mobile phase is Acetonitrile-water (25:75), and detection wavelength is 320nm. The number of theoretical plates of the column is not less than 2000, calculated with the reference to the peak of 2,3,5,4'-tetrahydroxystilbene-2-O-β-D-glucopyranoside.

3.2 Preparation of reference solution: Weigh accurately some of 2,3,5,4'-tetrahydroxystilbene-2-O-β-D-glucopyranoside and dissolve with ethanol to get the reference solution with the concentration of 0.2mg/mL.

3.3 Preparation of test solution: Weigh accurately 0.2g of the crude and processed drug samples in the conical flasks with cover respectively, and add 25mL of homeopathic alcohol. Weigh, heat to reflux for 0.5 hours, allow to cool, replenish the weight with homeopathic alcohol, mix well and filtrate.

3.4 Assay: Inject 10μL reference solution and test solution, record the peak area and determinate the content of the effective component.

◆ Experimental instruction

1. Preview

1.1 Which family and genus does Polygoni Multiflori Radix belong to? What about its function and taste? What are the changes of its function and taste after processing?

1.2 What effective ingredient does Polygoni Multiflori Radix contain? What functions do each of these ingredients have?

1.3 What synergistic actions do the drug and black bean have?

1.4 Review the principles of using the primary derivative spectrometry.

2. Primary operations and notes of the operations

2.1 Primary operations

2.1.1 Use Soxhlet's extractor correctly.

2.1.2 Use spectrophotometer and HPLC correctly.

2.2 Notes of the operations

2.2.1 No fire is permitted in the laboratory because of the use of organic solvents.

2.2.2 The processed drug must be smashed sufficiently, otherwise it will bring to bigger error.

2.2.3 Control the temperature strictly when using chloroform to extract and recover the solvent. The color error will appear when adding the solution at high temperature.

3. Format of the experimental report

3.1 Purpose

3.2 Principle

3.3 Experimental data and calculating results

Table 16-1 The results of anthrone assay in crude and processed drug

Sample	Weight (g)	A (free)	A (total)	Free (%)	Conjugate (%)	Total (%)
RPM						
RPMP						

Table 16-2 The results of diphenyl ethylenside assay in crude and processed drug

Sample	Weight (g)	A_{330}	A_{334}	ΔA	C (mg/mL)	Content (%)
RPM						
RPMP						

Table 16-3 The content of 2,3,5,4'-tetrahydroxystilbene-2-O-β-D-glucopyranoside

Sample	Weight (g)	Peak area	Concentration (μg/mL)	Content (%)
RPM				
RPMP				

3.4 Discussion

4. Considerations after the experiment

4.1 What are the processing methods for Polygoni Multiflori Radix? Why its purgative effect relieved after processing?

4.2 What are the quantitative determination methods for anthraquinones and astragalus in traditional Chinese medicine?

(Edited by De Ji and Yujiang Chen)

第六章 煮 法

实验十七 煮法的代表药物炮制

实验目的 •••

1. 掌握煮法的基本操作、注意事项及成品质量评价标准。
2. 掌握炮制辅料甘草水的制备方法。
3. 熟悉煮法的炮制目的和意义及辅料对药物作用的影响。

实验原理 •••

煮法可以使药物软化，便于切制，消除或降低药物的不良反应，缓和药性，增强疗效。

远志为远志科植物远志 *Polygala tenuifolia* Willd. 或卵叶远志 *Polygala sibirica* L. 的干燥根。具有安神益智、交通心肾、祛痰、消肿的功效。用于心肾不交引起的失眠多梦，健忘惊悸，神志恍惚，咳痰不爽，疮疡肿毒，乳房肿痛。远志生品"戟人咽喉"，多外用涂敷。甘草水煮后，既能缓和燥性，又能消除麻味，防止刺喉，以安神益智为主。

实验器材 •••

1. **仪器** 煮锅，电子秤，烧杯，搪瓷盘等。
2. **药材** 甘草，远志。

实验内容 •••

1. **甘草水的制备** 将甘草片置锅内加适量水煎煮两次（分别为30分钟和20分钟），过滤，合并滤液，再将甘草水浓缩至每10mL相当于1g甘草，备用。

2. **甘草水煮远志** 将净远志投入装有上述甘草水的锅内，加热煮沸，保持微沸，并勤翻动，至甘草水被吸尽，略干，取出干燥。每100kg远志，用甘草6kg。

实验指导 •••

1. 基本操作和操作注意点

（1）煮时用文火保持微沸，并勤翻动。辅料具有挥发性的，宜加盖煮制。

（2）甘草水制备时应浓缩至适宜浓度。

2. 实验报告格式

（1）实验目的

（2）实验原理

（3）实验内容

（4）讨论

3. 实验后思考

（1）简述甘草水制远志的炮制目的及注意事项。

（2）煮法炮制药物时，煮沸后为何需改用文火？

（马志国 孙小雅）

Experiment 17　Representative Medicinal Processing of Boiling Method

◆ Experimental purposes

1. To master the basic operations, precautions, and quality evaluation standards of boiling method.

2. To master the preparation method of Glycyrrhizae Radix et Rhizoma (Gancao) juice.

3. To understand the purpose and significance of boiling methods and the influence of excipients on drug action.

◆ Experimental principle

Boiling method can soften the drug and facilitate cutting, remove or decrease its toxicity and side effects, mitigate the property of drug and strengthen its curative effect.

Polygalae Radix is the dried root of *Polygala tenuifolia* Willd. or *Polygala sibirica* L. It can tranquilize the mind and replenish wisdom, dispel phlegm and disperse swelling. It can be used for insomnia and dreaminess caused by heart kidney disharmony, forgetfulness and palpitations, confusion, phlegm discomfort, sores and swelling, and breast pain. Raw Polygalae Radix is stimulating and for external use. After Glycyrrhizae Radix et Rhizoma juice boiling, it can relieve dryness and eliminate its numb taste, preventing the stinging of the throat. It is used primarily to calm the nerves and nourish the mind.

◆ Experimental apparatus

1. Instruments

Saucepan, Electronic scale, beaker, enamel tray, et al.

2. Medicinal materials

Polygalae Radix, Glycyrrhizae Radix et Rhizoma.

◆ Experimental content

1. Preparation of Glycyrrhizae Radix et Rhizoma juice

Boil Glycyrrhizae Radix et Rhizoma twice (30 minutes and 20 minutes respectively), filter and combine the filtrate, then concentrate the solution to the equivalent of 1g of Glycyrrhizae Radix et Rhizoma per 10mL and set aside.

2. Stir-baking Polygalae Radix with Glycyrrhizae Radix et Rhizoma juice

Mix drug with Glycyrrhizae Radix et Rhizoma juice, heat with mild fire, and boil until absorbed by drug entirely. Take them out and dry. For each 100kg of Glycyrrhizae Radix et Rhizoma, add 6kg Polygalae Radix.

◆ Experiment instruction

1. Primary operation and the notes of the operation

1.1 When boiling, keep it slightly boiling over low heat and stir frequently. If the excipients are volatile, they should be decocted with a cover.

1.2 Glycyrrhizae Radix et Rhizoma juice should be concentrated to the appropriate concentration during preparation.

2. Format of the experimental report

2.1 Purposes

2.2 Principle

2.3 The content of the experiment

2.4 Discussion

3. Considerations after the experiment

3.1 Briefly describe the processing purpose and precautions of stir-baking Polygalae Radix with Glycyrrhizae Radix et Rhizoma juice.

3.2 Why does it need to switch to low heat after boiling when decocting medicine?

（Edited by Zhiguo Ma and Xiaoya Sun）

实验十八　乌头的炮制及炮制前后生物碱的含量分析和毒性研究

实验目的 •••

1. 掌握乌头的炮制方法。
2. 掌握乌头中总生物碱及酯型生物碱的含量测定方法。
3. 掌握乌头的毒性实验方法。
4. 掌握乌头炮制前后生物碱类成分的质变与量变，以及这种变化与乌头毒性的关系，从而阐明乌头炮制的作用和意义。

实验原理 •••

乌头有川乌、草乌两种。川乌为毛茛科植物乌头 *Aconitum carmichaelii* Debx.的干燥母根，有祛风除湿、温经止痛的功效，用于风寒湿痹、关节疼痛、心腹冷痛、寒疝作痛及麻醉止痛。草乌为毛茛科植物北乌头 *Aconitum kusnezoffii* Reichb.的干燥块根，其性味、功效、用法、使用注意及炮制方法与川乌相似而毒性更强。

乌头具有极强的毒性，需炮制减毒后方可使用。其炮制方法据古今文献记载有70余种，现今主要有蒸、煮、黑豆甘草煮、生姜豆腐煮等。

乌头的毒性成分为二萜类双酯型生物碱，主要是乌头碱（aconitine）、新乌头碱（mesaconitine）、次乌头碱（hypaconitine）等。此类生物碱的毒性与C_8位和C_{14}位的酯键有关。乌头在浸漂和蒸煮过程中，由于生物碱类成分的流失和破坏，使其含量减少，毒性降低。乌头炮制减毒原理是双酯型生物碱，如乌头碱（aconitine）首先水解转变成为毒性较小的单酯型生物碱，如苯甲酰乌头原碱（benzoylaconitine）等，再进一步水解而转变成毒性更小的乌头原碱（aconine）等（以乌头碱为例其水解过程如图18-1所示）。此外，还有人提出另外一种炮制减毒原理，认为乌头碱类生物碱C_8位上的乙酰基，在比较缓和的加热条件下可以被一些长链脂肪酰基置换，从而生成毒性较小的脂乌头碱类（lipoaconitines）。

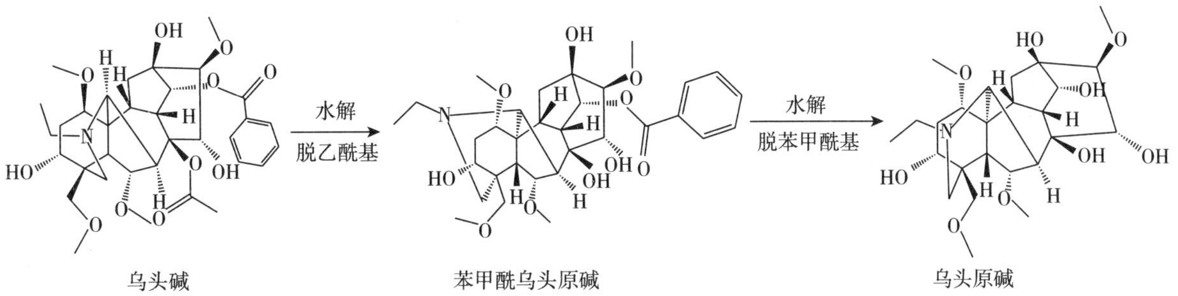

图18-1　乌头碱水解过程

由于乌头中总生物碱的含量与毒性强度没有平行关系，若只测定总碱含量并不能其评价毒性大小，只有分别测定双酯型生物碱和单酯型生物碱的总量才可控制其质量。因此本实验采用高效液相色谱法分别测定乌头及其炮制品中双酯型生物碱和单酯型生物碱的总量，并采用安全性实验来比较炮制前后的毒性差异。

实验器材 •••

1. 仪器　高效液相色谱仪，超声提取仪，旋转蒸发仪，水分测定仪，电热干燥箱，恒温水浴锅，分析天平，量筒，玻璃漏斗，具塞锥形瓶，蒸锅，高压灭菌锅，锅铲，煤气灶（或其他加热电器），搪瓷盘，切药刀，三号筛等。

2. 药材及试剂　乌头药材，乙腈，四氢呋喃，醋酸铵，冰醋酸，异丙醇，三氯甲烷，氨试液，乙酸乙酯，乌头碱对照品，次乌头碱对照品，新乌头碱对照品，苯甲酰乌头原碱对照品，苯甲酰次乌头原碱对照品，苯甲酰新乌头原碱对照品等。

实验内容 •••

1. 药材的炮制

（1）生乌头　取原药材，除去杂质，洗净干燥。

（2）煮乌头　取净乌头，大小个分开，用水浸泡至内无干心，取出，加水煮沸4~6小时（或蒸6~8小时）至取大个及实心者切开内无白心、口尝微有麻舌感时，取出，晾至六成干，切片，干燥。

（3）高压蒸乌头　取净乌头，放入高压灭菌锅内，锅压力为147.1kPa（1.5kg/cm²），热压50分钟，取出，晾干，切片，干燥。

2. 双酯型生物碱的含量测定

（1）色谱条件与系统适用性试验　以十八烷基硅烷键合硅胶为填充剂；以乙腈－四氢呋喃（25:15）为流动相A，以0.1mol/L醋酸铵溶液（每1000mL加冰醋酸0.5mL）为流动相B，按表18-1中的规定进行梯度洗脱；检测波长为235nm。

表18-1　梯度洗脱程序

时间（min）	流动相A（%）	流动相B（%）
0~48	15→26	85→74
48~49	26→35	74→65
49~58	35	65
58~65	35→15	65→85

（2）对照品溶液的制备　取乌头碱对照品、次乌头碱对照品及新乌头碱对照品适量，精密称定，加异丙醇－三氯甲烷（1:1）混合溶液分别制成每1mL含乌头碱50μg、次乌头碱和新乌头碱各0.15mg的混合溶液，即得。

（3）供试品溶液的制备　分别取生乌头、煮乌头和高压蒸乌头粉末（过三号筛）约2g，精密称定，置具塞锥形瓶中，加氨试液3mL，精密加入异丙醇－乙酸乙酯（1:1）混合溶液50mL，称定重量，超声处理（功率300W，频率40kHz；水温在25℃以下）30分钟，放冷，再称定重量，用异丙醇－乙酸乙酯（1:1）混合溶液补足减失的重量，摇匀，滤过。精密量取续滤液25mL，40℃以下减压回收溶剂至干，残渣精密加入异丙醇－三氯甲烷（1:1）混合溶液3mL溶解，滤过，取续滤液，即得。

（4）测定法　分别精密吸取对照品溶液与供试品溶液各10μL，注入液相色谱仪，测定，即得。按干燥品计，分别计算乌头不同炮制品中含乌头碱、次乌头碱、新乌头碱的百分含量。

3. 单酯型生物碱的含量测定

（1）色谱条件与系统适用性试验　同"2. 双酯型生物碱的含量测定"。

（2）对照品溶液的制备　取苯甲酰乌头原碱对照品、苯甲酰次乌头原碱对照品、苯甲酰新乌头原碱对照品适量，精密称定，加异丙醇–三氯甲烷（1∶1）混合溶液制成每1mL含苯甲酰乌头原碱和苯甲酰次乌头原碱各50μg、苯甲酰新乌头原碱0.3mg的混合溶液，即得。

（3）供试品溶液的制备　同"2. 双酯型生物碱的含量测定"。

（4）测定法　同"2. 双酯型生物碱的含量测定"。按干燥品计，分别计算乌头不同炮制品中含苯甲酰乌头原碱、苯甲酰次乌头原碱、苯甲酰新乌头原碱的百分含量。

4. 乌头炮制前后的毒性实验

（1）供试品溶液的制备　称取生乌头、煮乌头和高压蒸乌头粉末（过三号筛）各20g，加蒸馏水200mL，煮30分钟，过滤，残渣再煮两次，滤过，合并滤液，浓缩，均制成10%的样品液，滤过，备用。

（2）毒性实验　取体重18~22g小白鼠45只，随机分成3组，分别标号称重，然后以0.5mL/10g的剂量腹腔注射生乌头、煮乌头和高压蒸乌头样品液，观察2小时，记录动物中毒症状、死亡时间和死亡数目。

实验指导 •••

1. 预习

（1）蒸法、煮法的目的和含义各是什么？

（2）制乌头的炮制方法是什么？

（3）乌头双酯型生物碱和单酯型生物碱的含量测定方法是什么？

（4）乌头炮制前后的毒性实验方法是什么？

2. 基本操作和注意事项

（1）基本操作　①掌握生乌头、制乌头和高压蒸乌头的炮制方法。②掌握高效液相色谱法测定乌头双酯型生物碱的含量。③掌握高效液相色谱法测定乌头单酯型生物碱的含量。④掌握小鼠毒性实验方法。

（2）操作注意点　①乌头为剧毒药物，实验时要注意安全，在实验过程中应该严格进行管理，实验前领取药材及实验完毕交还制川乌时，均需称重量并进行登记，严禁私自处理。②毒性实验制备样品液时，需要在减压条件下或60℃水浴进行浓缩，以免在浓缩过程中乌头碱被破坏。

3. 实验报告格式

（1）实验目的

（2）实验原理

（3）实验内容及结果

①乌头的炮制

②双酯型和单酯型生物碱的含量测定

表18-2　乌头中双酯型和单酯型生物碱的含量测定

样品	样品重量（g）	双酯型生物碱含量（%）	单酯型生物碱含量（%）
生乌头			
煮乌头			
高压蒸乌头			

③ 小鼠毒性实验

表18-3　乌头炮制前后的小鼠毒性实验

样品	动物只数（只）	死亡时间（分钟）	死亡数（只）	死亡率（%）
生乌头				
煮乌头				
高压蒸乌头				

（4）讨论

4. 实验后思考

（1）乌头为什么要炮制？其炮制方法有哪些？

（2）根据本实验结果，你认为乌头的哪种炮制方法较好？理由是什么？

（3）为什么要分别测定乌头中双酯型和单酯型生物碱的含量？

（4）衡量乌头的毒性大小，除本实验方法外还有哪些方法？

（李兴华　孙小雅）

Experiment 18　The Determination of Alkaloid in Wutou (Aconiti Radix and Aconiti Kusnezoffii Radix) and the Toxic Test

◆ Experimental purposes

1. To master the different processing methods of Wutou.

2. To master the assaying method of total alkaloids and diester alkaloids.

3. To master the method of toxic test about Wutou.

4. Through this test, further understand the changes of alkaloids and the relationship between these changes and the toxicity of Wutou.

◆ Experimental principle

Wutou includes Aconiti Radix (chuan wu) and Aconiti Kusnezoffii Radix (cao wu) . Aconiti Radix (chuan wu) whose English name is commonly Monkshood Mother Root is the dried parent root tuber of *Aconitum carmichaelii* Debx. This drug can relieve rheumatic conditions and alleviate pain by warming the channels with the indications of joint pain in rheumatic or rheumatoid arthritis, epigastric pain with cold sensation, or abdominal colic due to cold, also it can be used as an analgesic in anaesthesia and so on. Aconti Kusnezoffii Radix (cao wu), Kusnzoff Monkshood Root, is the dried root tuber of *Aconitum Kusnezoffii* Reichb. Although its characters, actions, processing, usage, dosage and precaution are similar to that of chuan wu, the toxicity of cao wu is much stronger.

Since Wutou has a dramatic toxicity, it only can be used after being processed. More than 70 kinds of processing methods of Wutou are reported in the books and journals. But recently, we usually use steaming, boiling, boiling with black bean and glycyrhizia, and boiling with bean curd and fresh ginger and so on.

The toxic components of Wutou are diester alkaloids including aconitine, mesaconitine, hypaconitine and so on. The toxicity of this kind of alkaloids is related to the ester-bond in the position of C_8 and C_{14}. Through the procedure of macerating and steaming, the content and the toxicity of alkaloids decrease due to the decomposition of alkaloids.

The principle of reducing toxicity of processed Wutou is that the diester alkaloids first change into the single ester alkaloids, which has the small toxicity through hydrolysis, then lose the benzyl and hydrolysis to aconitines, which has the smallest toxicity. In addition, someone proposed another processing principle, and thought that the acetat C_8 of aconitines was replaced by long-chain lipo-acyl under the slowly mild heating conditions to turn into lipo-aconitines. Here is the hydrolysis of aconitines:

aconitine　　　　　　　　benzoylaconine　　　　　　　　aconine

HPLC is used to determine the content of diester aconitine and benzoylmonoester alkaloids indifferent processed products of Wutou.

◆ Instruments and apparatus

1. Instruments

High performance liquid chromatograph, ultrasonic extractor, rotary vaporizer, moisture tester, electric drying oven, constant temperature water bath steamer, truner, electric heater, enamel tray, herb cutting knife, No.3 sieve, etc.

2. Medicinal materials and chemicals

Wutou, Aconitine reference sample, Hypaconitine reference sample, Mesaconitine reference sample, Benzoylaconitine reference sample, Benzoylhypacoitine reference sample, Benzoylmesaconine reference sample, acetonitrile, tetrahydrofuran, ammonium acetate, ethanol, ammonia water, isopropanol, trichloromethane, ethyl acetate, glacial aceticacid, redistilled water, etc.

◆ Experimental content

1. Processing of drug

1.1 Wutou: Remove the foreign matters, break to pieces before using.

1.2 Boiling Wutou: Separate clean Aconiti Radix and Aconiti Kusnezoffii Radix by size, macerate in water thoroughly until there is no dry core. Then, take them out and boil in water for 4 to 6 hours (or steam 6 to 8 hours) until there is no white core in the relatively large and solid root and the taste becomes slightly numb. After removal, dry in the air, cut into slices, dry again.

1.3 Steaming Wutou over high pressure: Put the clean Aconiti Radix and Aconiti Kusnezoffii Radix in high pressure cooker (147.1kPa, 1.5kg/cm^2), and heat for 50 minutes, take out and dry.

2. Determination of the diester alkaloids

2.1 Chromatographic system and systematic adaptation test: Use octadecylsilane bonded silica gel as the stationary phase, a mixture of acetonitrile and tetrahydrofuran (25 : 15) as the mobile phase A and a 0.1mol/L solution of ammonium acetate (add 0.5mL glacial acetic acid in each 1000mL solution) as the mobile phase B, gradient elution procedures are shown in table. As detection wavelength set at 235nm, the number of theoretical plates of the column shall not be less than 2000.

Table 18-1   Gradient elution procedures

Time (min)	Mobile phase A (%)	Mobile phase B (%)
0~48	15→26	85→74
48~49	26→35	74→65
49~58	35	65
58~65	35→15	65→85

2.2 Preparation of reference sample solution: Weigh accurately appropriate amount of aconitine, hypaconitine and mesaconitine references ample, respectively, and dissolve them. Add isopropanol-chloroform （ 1 : 1 ）mixture to produce a mixed solution containing 50μg of aconitine, 0.15mg each of hypaconitine and mesaconitine per 1mL.

2.3 Preparation of test sample solution: Weigh accurately 2g of processed product powder (passing sieve

No.3), put into a conical flask with plug, add 3ml of ammonia test solution, accurately add 50ml of a mixture of isopropanol and ethylacetate (1∶1) and weigh. Ultrasonicate (power 300W, frequency 40kHz, keeping the water temperature below 25℃) 30 minutes, allow to cool and weigh again, replenish the weight loss of the solvent with the above mixture, mix well and filter. Measure accurately 25mL of the subsequent filtrate, recover the solvent to dryness in vacuum below 40℃, dissolve the residue in 3ml of the above mixture, filter and use the subsequent filtrate as the test sample solution.

2.4 Determination method: Accurately pipette 10μL of the reference sample solution and the test sample solution respectively into the column, and calculate the content. According to the dry products, the percentage contents of aconitine, hypaconitine and mesaconitine in different processed products of Wutou are calculated.

3. Determination of benzoylmonoester alkaloids in different processed products of Wutou

3.1 Chromatographic conditions and system atic adaptation test: The same as the method of "2. Determination of the diester alkaloids" .

3.2 Preparation of reference sample solution: Weigh accurately appropriate amount of Benzoylaconine, Benzoylhypacoitine and Benzoylmesaconine, respectively, then dissolve. Add the mixture of isopropanol and chloroform (1∶1) to produce a mixed solution containing 50μg each of Benzoylaconine and Benzoylhypacoitine, 0.3mg of Benzoylmesaconine per 1mL.

3.3 Preparation of test sample solution: The same as the method of "2. Determination of the diester alkaloids" .

3.4 Determination method: The same as the method of "2. Determination of the diester alkaloids" . According to the dry products, the percentage contents of Benzoylaconine, Benzoylhypacoitine and Benzoylmesaconine in different processed products of Wutou are calculated.

4. Experiment of the toxicity of raw and processed Wutou (Aconitti)

4.1 Preparation of sample solution: Weigh accurately 20g crude (unprocessed) Wutou, steamed Wutou under high pressure and boiled Wutou respectively, add 200mL steamed water, boil for 30 minutes, and filter. Boil the residue with water for 2 times, filter again. Combine the filtrates and concentrate to a 10% sample solution, filter to use.

4.2 Toxic experiment: Divide randomly 45 little mice with the weight ranging from 18 to 22g into 3 groups. Weigh and indicate them respectively, then intraperitoneal inject the three kinds of sample solution with the dosage of 0.5mL/10g, observe them for 2 hours, record their intoxication symptoms, the time and the number of their death.

◆ Experimental instruction

1. Preview

1.1 Learn about the goals of steaming and boiling.

1.2 Familiarize the processing methods of Wutou.

1.3 Master the assaying methods of diester alkaloids and benzoylmonoester alkaloids.

1.4 Learn about the methods of toxic experiment.

2. Primary operations and notes of the operations

2.1 Primary operations

2.1.1 Master the methods of processing of Wutou.

2.1.2 Master the methods of assaying the diester alkaloids.

2.1.3 Master the methods of assaying the benzoylmonoester alkaloids.

2.1.4 Master the methods of toxic experiment on mice.

2.2 Notes of operations

2.2.1 Pay attention to safety because of the dramatic toxicity of Wutou. Wutou is a kind of toxic traditional Chinese medicine. Therefore, it should be strictly managed during the experiment. Before the experiment, when receiving the medicine and returning the processed Wutou and raw Chinese medicine after the experiment, they should be weighed and registered. It is strictly prohibited to handle without permission.

2.2.2 Better to concentrate the solution under vacuum conditions or 60℃ water bath, when preparing the sample solutions for toxic experiment, so as to avoid destroying the aconitine.

3. Format of the experimental report

3.1 Purpose

3.2 Principle

3.3 Experimental data and calculating results

3.3.1 The processing of Wutou

3.3.2 The content of ester alkaloids

Table 18-2　The content of ester alkaloids

Sample	Weight (g)	Diester alkaloids (%)	Benzoylmonoester alkaloids (%)
Raw Wutou			
Boiled Wutou			
Steamed Wutou over pressure			

3.3.3 Toxic experiment on mice

Table 18-3　Toxic experiment on mice

Sample	Number of mice	Time to death (min)	Number of death	Death rate (%)
Raw Wutou				
Boiled Wutou				
Steamed Wutou over pressure				

3.3.4 Discussion

4. Considerations after the experiment

4.1 Why should Wutou be processed? How many processing methods of it are there?

4.2 Which method do you think is better according to the experimental data? Why?

4.3 Why should we assay the ester-alkaloids? Is it just right to assay the total alkaloids only?

4.4 What other methods are there besides the one used in this experiment to evaluate the toxicity of Wutou?

(Edited by Xinghua Li and Xiaoya Sun)

第七章　燀　法

实验十九　燀法的代表药物炮制

实验目的 ●•

1. 掌握燀苦杏仁的炮制方法、注意事项及成品质量评价标准。
2. 熟悉苦杏仁燀制的目的和意义。

实验原理 ●•

苦杏仁味苦，性微温，有小毒。归肺、大肠经。具有降气止咳平喘、润肠通便的功能。生品性微温而质润，长于润肺止咳，润肠通便。多用于新病喘咳，肠燥便秘。燀制可破坏苦杏仁苷酶，保存苦杏仁苷；并除去非药用部位，便于有效成分煎出，提高药效。

实验器材 ●•

1. 仪器　蒸锅，电子秤，烧杯，搪瓷盘等。
2. 药材　苦杏仁等。

实验内容 ●•

燀苦杏仁　取净苦杏仁置10倍量沸水中，加热约5分钟，至种皮微膨起即捞出，用凉水浸泡，取出，搓开种皮与种仁，干燥，筛去种皮。用时捣碎。

实验指导 ●•

1. 基本操作和操作注意点

（1）燀制用水量一般为药材重量的10倍以上。若水量少，投入药物后水温迅速降低，酶不能很快被灭活，反而使苷被酶解，影响药效。

（2）水沸腾后投入药物，加热时间以5～10分钟为宜。若燀制时间过长，易导致成分损失。

（3）燀去皮后宜当天晒干或低温烘干，否则易泛油，色变黄，影响成品质量。

2. 实验报告格式

（1）实验目的
（2）实验原理
（3）实验内容
（4）讨论

3. 实验后思考

如何判断苦杏仁燀制时的杀酶保苷效果？

（李兴华　陆奕霜）

Experiment 19　Representative Medicinal Processing of Blanching

◆ Experimental purposes

1. To master the basic operations, precautions, and quality evaluation standards of blanching methods.

2. To understand the purpose and significance of blanching Armeniacae Semen Amarum.

◆ Experimental principle

Armeniacae Semen Amarum is bitter in flavor, mildly warm in property, small in toxicity, lungand and large intestine in channel tropism. It has the functions of relieving cough and asthma and relaxing bowel for cough phlegm, constipation due to intestinal dryness, etc. The activity of the amygdalase is destroyed by blanching processing and the amygdalin is preserved, safety and effectiveness of clinical application are guaranteed.

◆ Instruments and medicinal materials

1. Instruments

Stainless steel pot, counter balance, beaker, enamel tray, et al.

2. Medicinal materials

Armeniacae Semen Amarum, et al.

◆ Experimental content

Blanching

Armeniacae Semen Amarum (Kuxingren)

Put the cleaning Armeniacae Semen Amarum into boiling water whose quantity is 10 times as much as Armeniacae Semen Amarum, heat for about 5 minutes until the testa is slightly swollen, then scoopit up, soak it in cold water, take it out, rub the testa and kernel, make it dry, and sieve the testa. Mash it when used.

◆ Experiment instruction

1. Primary operation and the notes of the operation

1.1 Quantity of water for blanching should be more than ten times of the drug. If the quantity of water is low, the enzyme cannot be destroyed.

1.2 Time for blanching should be five to ten minutes. If the time is too long, the amygdalin will be lost.

1.3 It is better to dry in the sun or at a low-temperature intraday. Otherwise, it may cause oil spillage, turn yellow, and affect the quality of the finished product.

2. Format of the experimental report

2.1 Purposes

2.2 Principle

2.3 The content of the experiment

2.4 Discussion

3. Considerations after the experiment

How to determine the enzyme killing and amygdalin protecting effect of blanching of Armeniacae Semen Amarum?

（ Edited by Xinghua Li and Yishuang Lu ）

实验二十　苦杏仁及其炮制品中苦杏仁苷的定性、定量分析

实验目的 ●●●

1.掌握苦杏仁及其炮制品中苦杏仁苷的定性、定量分析方法。

2.通过对苦杏仁及其炮制品中苦杏仁苷的定性、定量分析，了解苦杏仁炮制的目的及其原理。

实验原理 ●●●

苦杏仁为蔷薇科植物山杏 *Prunus armeniaca* L.var.ansu Maxim.、西伯利亚杏 *Prunus sibirica* L.、东北杏 *Prunus mandshurica*（Maxim.）Koehne 或杏 *Prunus armeniaca* L. 的干燥成熟种子。具有降气止咳平喘，润肠通便的功效，用于咳嗽气喘、胸闷痰多、肠燥便秘。苦杏仁中的止咳平喘主要有效成分是苦杏仁苷（amygdalin），口服苦杏仁后，其中苦杏仁苷经胃酸的作用在体内缓缓分解而产生微量的氢氰酸，起到镇静呼吸中枢作用而达止咳平喘之效。但苦杏仁中含有苦杏仁苷酶（amygdalase），能使苦杏仁苷水解成野樱苷（prunasin）。野樱苷能继续被野樱苷酶（prunase）水解，生成杏仁腈。杏仁腈性不稳定，遇热易分解生成苯甲醛（有典型的杏仁香味）和氢氰酸。其酶解过程如下：

燀法炮制能破坏苦杏仁酶的活性，增加苦杏仁苷的稳定性，保证用药安全有效。本实验利用苦味酸钠试验（生品中苦杏仁苷被苦杏仁酶水解生成氰氢酸，接触苦味酸钠试纸发生还原反应，生成异紫酸钠显砖红色，而炮制品则不显砖红色），定性检测苦杏仁中酶的活性。同时采用高效液相色谱法进行苦杏仁苷的含量测定。

实验器材 ●●●

1. 仪器　高效液相色谱仪，烧杯，量筒，研钵，具塞试管，恒温水浴锅，超声波清洗仪，分析天平等。

2. 药材及试剂 苦杏仁，苦味酸钠试纸，甲醇，乙腈，磷酸等。

实验内容 •••

1. 苦杏仁苷的定性分析 取捣碎后的生苦杏仁、燀苦杏仁和炒苦杏仁样品约0.5g，分别置试管中，加水数滴使湿润，在试管口悬挂一条苦味酸钠试纸，管口用软木塞塞紧，将试管置40~50℃水浴中加热，观察试纸的颜色变化。

2. 苦杏仁苷的含量测定

色谱条件与系统适用性试验 以十八烷基硅烷键合硅胶为填充剂；以乙腈–0.1%磷酸溶液（8∶92）为流动相；检测波长为207nm。理论板数按苦杏仁苷峰计算应不低于7000。

对照品溶液的制备 取苦杏仁苷对照品适量，精密称定，加甲醇制成每1mL含40μg的溶液，即得。

供试品溶液的制备 分别取生苦杏仁、燀苦杏仁和炒苦杏仁粉末（过二号筛）约0.25g，精密称定，置具塞锥形瓶中，精密加入甲醇25mL，密塞，称定重量，超声处理（功率250W，频率50kHz）30分钟，放冷，再称定重量，用甲醇补足减失的重量，摇匀，滤过，精密量取续滤液5mL，置50mL量瓶中，加50%甲醇稀释至刻度，摇匀，滤过，取续滤液，即得。

测定法 分别精密吸取对照品溶液与供试品溶液各10~20μL，注入液相色谱仪，测定，即得。

实验指导 •••

1. 预习 苦杏仁苷的定性分析方法和含量测定方法是什么？

2. 基本操作和操作注意点

（1）基本操作 掌握苦杏仁及其炮制品中苦杏仁苷的定性、定量分析方法。

（2）操作注意点 炒制苦杏仁的火候对苦杏仁苷含量的影响很大，用文火炒至微黄、略有焦斑为宜，忌将苦杏仁炒黑炒炭。

3. 实验报告格式

（1）实验目的

（2）实验原理

（3）实验内容及结果

① 苦杏仁苷的定性分析

表20-1 苦味酸钠实验

样品	加热时间（min）	颜色变化
生苦杏仁		
燀苦杏仁		
炒苦杏仁		

② 苦杏仁苷的定量分析

表20-2 苦杏仁苷含量

样品	样品重量（g）	苦杏仁苷含量（%）
生苦杏仁		
燀苦杏仁		
炒苦杏仁		

（4）讨论

4. 实验后思考

（1）苦杏仁苷可被苦杏仁苷酶或酸水解，且不同水解条件可得到不同的水解产物。若分别用苦杏仁苷酶、稀酸、浓酸水解药材中的苦杏仁苷，试回答它们的水解过程和水解产物应是什么？

（2）测定苦杏仁中苦杏仁苷的含量，有哪几种方法？

（3）你认为哪种炮制方法能使苦杏仁中的苦杏仁苷损失最小？

（李兴华 陆奕霜）

Experiment 20 Processing of and Qualitative and Quantitative Analysis of the Crude and the Processed Armeniacae Semen Amarum

◆ Experimental purpose

1. To master the qualitative and quantitative analysis of amygdalin.

2. To understand the aim and principle of Armeniacae Semen Amarum by qualitative and quantitative analysis of amygdalin and its processed drug.

◆ Experimental principle

Armeniacae Semen Amarum is the dried ripe seed of *Prunus armeniaca* L.var.ansu Maxim., *Prunus sibirica* L., *Prunus mandshurica* (Maxim.) Koehne or *Prunus armeniaca* L. (Fam. Rosaceae), which can relieve cough and asthma, and relax bowels. It can be used to cure cough and asthma accompanied by stuffiness in the chest and profuse expectoration; constipation due to deficiency of blood and fluid. Its active component to relieve cough and asthma is amygdalin. After taking it orally, it can be slowly decomposed and produce little hydrocyanic acid which can sedate respiration center and relieve cough and asthma, in the circumstance of the acid in stomach. However, there is amygdalase in Armeniacae Semen Amarum, which can hydrolyze amygdalin into prunasin that can also be decomposed into acid nitrile of almond in the existence of prunase. While the acid nitrile of almond is instable and easily decomposed into benzaldehyde (with characteristic odor of almond) and acid nitrile of almond. The following is the process of enzymatic hydrolysis:

Boiling in water can destroy amygdalase and increase the stability of amygdalin, and ensure the safety and effectiveness of medication. In this experiment, we take the sodium test (amygdalin in raw products is hydrolyzed by amygdalase to produce hydrocyanic acid, which is reduced by contact with the sodium picrate test paper to produce sodium isocyanurate that shows brick red, while processed products do not show brick red) to qualitatively detect the enzyme activity in Armeniacae Semen Amarum. At the same time, the content of amygdalin is determined by HPLC.

$$\text{trinitrophenol} + 2NaCN \longrightarrow \text{brick-red} + NaCNO$$

◆ Experimental apparatus

1. Instruments

The equipment of HPLC, sieve, beaker, measuring cylinder, mortar, test tube with a stopper, thermostatic water bath, ultrasonic cleaner, electronic balance, etc.

2. Medicinal materials and chemicals

Armeniacae Semen Amarum, sodium picrate test paper, methanol, acetonitrile, phosphoric acid, etc.

◆ Experimental content

1. Identification

Sodium picrate test: Break several grains of the drug to pieces and immediately place about 0.5g into a test tube, moisten with several drops of water, hang a strip of trinitrophenol TP and plug the nozzle tightly with a cork. Heat on a warm water bath at 40-50℃, observe the color of the test paper.

2. Determination of amygdalin

2.1 Chromatographic conditions and systematic adaptation test: Samples are analyzed on the C_{18} reversed phase chromatography column with the mobile phase consisted of acetonitrile-0.1% phosphoric acid (8 : 92). The detection wavelength is set at 207nm. The number of theoretical plates of the column shall be no less than 7000.

2.2 Preparation of reference sample solution: Weigh an appropriate amount of amygdalin reference sample accurately and add methanol to prepare an amygdalin reference substance sample solution with a mass concentration of 40μg/mL.

2.3 Preparation of test sample solution: Weigh accurately the crude and processed Armeniacae Semen Amarum (passed through a No.2 sieve) about 0.25g accurately, place them in a conical flask with a plug, add 25mL of methanol and then weigh them. Ultrasonication (power 250W, frequency 50kHz) for 30 minutes, allow to cool, weigh again, replenish the weight loss with methanol, mix well, filter, take 5mL of the subsequent filtrate and pour it in a 50mL volumetric flask, add 50% methanol to the mark, mix well and filter to obtain the test sample solution.

2.4 Method of determination: Accurately pipette 10-20μL of each solution for analysisand determination. Based on the dried product, calculate the percentage of amygdalin in different processed products of Armeniacae Semen Amarum.

◆ Experimental instruction

1. Preview

Identification and determination of amygdalin.

2. Primary operations and notes of the operations

2.1 Primary operations

Grasp the method of identification of cyanogenic glycoside and determination of amygdalin.

2.2 Notes of the operations

For the stir-fried Armeniacae Semen Amarum, the duration and degree of heating have big influence on the content of hydrocyanic acid. Fry the drug with gentle heat until slight yellow rather than black color.

3. Format of the experimental report

3.1 Purpose

3.2 Principle

3.3 Experiment data and calculation results

3.3.1 Sodium picrate test

Table 20-1　Sodium picrate test

Sample	Time span of heating (min)	Variations of color
Crude Armeniacae Semen Amarum		
Blanched Armeniacae Semen Amarum		
Stir-fired Armeniacae Semen Amarum		

3.3.2 Content of amygdalin

Table 20-2　Content of amygdalin

Sample	Weight of sample (g)	Content of amygdalin (%)
Crude Armeniacae Semen Amarum		
Blanched Armeniacae Semen Amarum		
Stir-fired Armeniacae Semen Amarum		

3.4 Discussion

4. Considerations after the experiment

4.1 Amygdalin can be hydrolyzed by amygdalase or acid and different conditions derive different products. If we hydrolyze amygdalin by dilute acid, concentrated acid and amygdalase, what are the processes and products of hydrolysis separately?

4.2 How many means are there to determinate the content of amygdalin?

4.3 Which is the best processing method of losing the least amygdalin during processing?

(Edited by Xinghua Li and Yishuang Lu)

第八章　其他制法

实验二十一　其他制法的代表药物炮制

实验目的 •••

1. 掌握提净法、水飞法、发芽法、发酵法、制霜法、煨法、干馏法的基本操作方法、注意事项及饮片质量要求。

2. 了解提净法、水飞法、发芽法、发酵法、制霜法、煨法、干馏法的目的和意义。

实验原理 •••

提净法主要针对某些矿物药，特别是一些可溶性无机盐类药物，经过溶解、过滤、除净杂质后，再进行重结晶，以进一步纯净药物的方法。

水飞法主要针对某些不溶于水的矿物药，是利用粗细粉末在水中悬浮性不同，将不溶于水的矿物、贝壳类药物反复研磨，而分离制备极细腻粉末的方法。

通过发芽，淀粉被分解为糊精、葡萄糖和单糖，蛋白质被降解成为氨基酸，脂肪被分解成为甘油和脂肪酸，并产生各种消化酶类、维生素等，使药效物质基础发生改变，改变药物原有性能，使其具有新的功效，扩大用药品种。

发酵过程主要是利用微生物自身产生的酶系对药物的营养成分进行利用和代谢形成各种代谢产物，从而使药物可以产生新的功效。

生巴豆毒性强烈，仅供外用，其毒性成分主要包含在巴豆油中，去油制霜后能去除大部分的脂肪油，从而降低毒性，缓和峻泻作用。

煨法可以降低药物不良反应，增强疗效，缓和药性。

干馏法是将药物置于容器内，以火烤灼，使产生汁液的方法。制备有别于原药材的干馏物，以适合临床需要。

实验器材 •••

1. 仪器　蒸锅，漏水容器，电磁炉，天平，煮锅，吸水草纸，压榨器，研钵，磁铁。

2. 药材　萝卜，朴硝，朱砂，滑石粉，黑大豆，桑叶，青蒿，巴豆，肉豆蔻，麦麸，鸡蛋。

实验内容 •••

1. 提净法

芒硝　取适量鲜萝卜，洗净，切成片，置煮制容器内，加适量水煮透，捞出萝卜，再投入适量天然芒硝（朴硝）共煮，至全部溶化，取出澄清以后取上清液，放冷。待结晶大部析出，取出置避风处适当干燥即得。其结晶母液经浓缩后可继续析出结晶，至不再析出结晶为止。每100kg朴硝，用萝卜20kg。

2. 水飞法

（1）朱砂　取原药材，用磁铁吸尽铁屑，置研钵内，加适量清水研磨成糊状，然后加多量清水搅拌，倾出混悬液，下沉的粗粉再如上法，反复操作，直至手捻细腻，无闪亮星为止，弃去杂质，合并混悬液，静置后倾去上面的清水，取沉淀晾干或40℃以下干燥，再研细，即得。

（2）滑石粉　取净滑石粗粉，加少量水，研磨至细，再加适量清水搅拌，倾出混悬液，下沉的粗粉再如上法，反复操作，合并混悬液，静置后倾去上面的清水，取沉淀干燥后再研细，即得。

3. 发芽法

大豆黄卷　取净大豆，用水浸泡至膨胀，倾去水，用湿布覆盖，每日淋水二次，待芽长至0.5～1cm时，取出，干燥。

4. 发酵法

淡豆豉　取桑叶、青蒿各70～100 g，加水煎煮，滤过，煎液拌入1000g净大豆中，吸尽后，蒸透，取出，稍晾，再置容器内，用煎过的桑叶、青蒿渣覆盖，闷使发酵至黄衣上遍时，取出，除去药渣，洗净，置容器内再闷15～20天，至充分发酵、香气溢出时，取出，略蒸，干燥，即得。

5. 制霜法

巴豆霜　取净巴豆仁，碾成泥状，布包严，蒸至圆汽30分钟。取出，压榨去油，再蒸再压。反复几次，至药物松散成粉末，不再粘结成饼为度。或取净巴豆仁碾细，测定脂肪油含量，加适量淀粉稀释，使脂肪油含量符合规定，混匀，即得。

6. 煨法

麦麸煨肉豆蔻　将麦麸和净肉豆蔻同置预热的炒制容器内，用文火加热并适当翻动，至麦麸呈焦黄色，肉豆蔻呈深棕色时取出，筛去麦麸，放凉，即得。

每100kg药物，用麦麸40kg。

7. 干馏法

蛋黄馏油　鸡蛋煮熟后，剥取蛋黄置适当容器内，以文火加热，除尽水分后用武火炒熬，至蛋黄油出尽为止，滤尽蛋黄油装瓶备用。

实验指导 •••

1. 预习

（1）发酵法、发芽法的适宜温湿度条件是什么？

（2）发酵法、发芽法制备药物的目的是什么？

（3）巴豆制霜时应该注意的问题有哪些？

（4）干馏法的炮制目的有哪些？

2. 基本操作和操作注意点

（1）提净法制备芒硝时加水要适量，以免影响结晶。水飞研磨过程中，水量宜少，搅拌混悬时加水量宜大，以除去有毒物质或杂质。

（2）朱砂干燥时温度不宜过高，以晾干为宜。

（3）发酵法、发芽法均须控制温度和湿度。一般发酵时空气的相对湿度应控制在70%~80%；发酵的最佳温度为30~37℃，发芽法一般以18~25℃为宜。

（4）原料在发酵前应进行杀菌、杀虫的处理，以免杂菌影响发酵质量。

（5）发酵过程必须一次完成，不能中断，或中途停顿。发酵品要芳香无霉味、酸败味。

（6）发芽时应该避光，勤加检查、淋水，保持相应的湿度，防止发热霉烂。

（7）原料不同，制备干馏物所需温度不同。

3. 实验报告格式

（1）实验目的

（2）实验原理

（3）实验内容

（4）讨论

4. 实验后思考

（1）芒硝提净过程中萝卜的作用是什么？

（2）发酵法、发芽法的原理是什么？

（3）发芽中为什么要控制适宜的芽长？

（4）煨法与固体辅料炒的异同点？

（杨小林　马志国　孙小雅）

Experiment 21   The Processing of Representative Drug of Other Preparation Methods

◆ Experimental purposes

1. To master the basic processing methods, precautions and quality requirements of purification, levigation, germination, fermentation, frost-like powder making, roasting, dry-distillation.

2. To understand the processing purpose and significance of purification, levigation, germination, fermentation, frost-like powder making, roasting, dry-distillation.

◆ Experimental principle

The purification method is mainly directed at some mineral medicines, especially some soluble inorganic salt drugs. After dissolution, filtration, and impurity removal, the drug is further purified by recrystallization.

Some water-insoluble mineral medicine, whose coarse and fine powder have different suspension properties in water. According to this property, the method of separating and preparing water-insoluble minerals and shellfish drug by repeated grinding to make extremely fine powder is called levigating.

Through germination, starch is decomposed into dextrin, glucose, and monosaccharide, protein is degraded into amino acids, and fats are hydrolyzed into glycerol and fatty acids, producing various digestive enzymes, vitamins, etc., changing the material basis of the drug effect and altering the original properties of the drug to develop new efficacy and expand the variety of medications.

The fermentation process mainly uses the enzymes produced by microorganisms themselves to utilize and metabolize the nutritional components of the drug to form various metabolites, so that it can produce new effects.

The raw croton fruit is hypertoxic, and can be only used externally. The croton oil is the main toxic component of the drug, and frosting by defatting can remove most croton oil to reduce toxicity and moderates purgative action.

The roasting method can reduce the side effects of the drug, enhance its efficacy and moderate its medicinal properties.

The dry-distillation is a method in which the drug is placed in a container and roasted over a fire to produce liquids. A dry distillate different from the original herb is prepared to suit clinical needs.

◆ Experimental apparatus

1. Instruments

Steamer, leaky container, induction cooker, balance, cooking pot, absorbent herb paper, squeezer, mortar, magnet etc.

2. Medicinal materials

Radish, mirabilite, cinnabar, talc, soybean, Folium Mori, Herba Artemisiae, Crotonis Fructus, Myristicae Semen, wheat bran, eggs.

◆ Experimental content

1. Purification method

Mirabilite (Mangxiao)

Cut the cleaned fresh radish into pieces, boil with water, take out the radish, and then put in a suitable amount of natural mirabilite, heat until the mirabilite dissolved, filter or take the supernatant after clarification, and let it cool. When the crystals are mostly precipitated, take it out and put it in a sheltered place to dry properly. The crystalline mother liquor can continue to precipitate crystals after concentration until no more crystals are precipitated.

Use 20 kg of fresh radish for every 100kg of mirabilite.

2. Levi gation method

2.1 Cinnabar (Zhusha)

Take the raw cinnabar, use the magnet to absorb all iron filings, put in a mortar, add an appropriate amount of water, grind them into paste, then add a large amount of water to stir, and pour out the suspension. Repeat the above operation several times for the sinking coarse powder, until it twists fine and there is no bright star. Discard the impurities, merge the suspension, pour out the top water after standing, take the precipitation to dry by airing, and grind fine. Or use magnet to remove iron filings in cinnabar, use ball mill to grand into fine powder with water. Oven dry below 40℃ and pass through the sieve with 200 meshes per square inch.

2.2 Talc (Huashi)

Take clean talc coarse powder, add a small amount of water and grind until fine. Add an appropriate amount of water and stir, then pour out the suspension. The sinking coarse powder should be repeatedly operated as above multiple times. Combine the suspension, let it stand, and then pour out the clean water on top. Take the sediment and dry it before grinding it fine to obtain it.

3. Germination method

Sojae Semen Germinatum (Dadouhuangjuan)

Take net soybeans, soak them in water until swell, put away the water, cover them with a wet cloth, drench them twice a day, wait for the buds to grow to 0.5-1cm, take them out, and dry them.

4. Fermentation method

Sojae Semen Praeparatum (Dandouchi)

Weigh Folium Mori and Herba Artemisiae Annuae 70-100g separately. Add in water and decoct. Filter and liquid medicine, then mix in 1000g soybean. Absorb completely and steam. Take out and cool a little. Cover soybean with dregs of decoction of Folium Mori and Herba Artemisiae Annuae, then put them in the incubator. Ferment for 6-8 days until "yellow clothes" overgrow, then take out and remove dregs of decoction. Wash cleanly and dry. Put them in the incubator that closed tightly for 15-20 days. Take out and steam to dryness.

5. Frost-like powder making method

Crotonis Semen Pulveratum (Badoushuang)

Take clean Crotonis Fructus, remove the shell, grind it into a mud shape, wrap it tightly, steam it for 30 minutes. Remove, press to remove oil, steam and press again. Repeat above procedure several times, until the drug loose into powder, no longer bonded into the cake for degree, or take the net Crotonis Fructus kernel to grind fine, determine the content of croton oil, add appropriate amount of starch dilution, make the content of croton oil in accordance with the provisions, and mix.

6. Roasting method

Myristicae Semen roasted in wheat bran (Maifuweiroudoukou)

Put the nutmeg and wheat bran into the pot together, heat with mild fire and stir properly. Take them out while the wheat bran becomes scorched yellow and the nutmegs become dark brown. Sift out the wheat bran and cool.

40kg of wheat bran is used for every 100kg of nutmegs.

7. Dry-distillation method

Egg yolk distillation oil (Danhuangliuyou)

After the egg is boiled, peel the yolk and place it in a suitable container, heat it with mild fire, remove the water and then scramble it with a strong fire until the yolk oil is exhausted, strain the oil and bottle it.

◆ Experimental instruction

1. Preview

1.1 What are the suitable temperature and humidity conditions for the fermentation and germination methods?

1.2 What is the purpose of fermentation and germination methods for preparing drug?

1.3 What are the problems that should be noted when making Crotonis Semen Pulveratum?

1.4 What are the processing purposes of the dry-distillation method?

2. Primary operation and the notes of the operation

2.1 When preparing mirabilite by purification method, water should be added in appropriate amount to avoid affecting the crystallization. It should add a small amount of water in the process of grinding but more water in the process of stirring and suspending to remove toxic substances or impurities with low solubility.

2.2 The drying temperature of cinnabar should not be too high; it is better to dry by airing.

2.3 Fermentation method and germination method require to control temperature and humidity. Generally, the relative humidity of the air should be controlled at 70%-80% during fermentation, the optimal temperature for fermentation is 30-37℃. The suitable temperature for germination is generally between 18-25℃.

2.4 Raw materials should be sterilized and insecticidal treatment before fermentation to avoid miscellaneous bacteria affecting the quality of fermentation.

2.5 The fermentation process must be completed at one time, without interruption or stopping in the middle. Fermented products should be aromatic without moldy and sour smell.

2.6 During germination, it should be kept in a dark place, checked and watered frequently, maintaining appropriate humidity to prevent heating and rotting.

2.7 Different raw materials require different temperatures for the preparation of dry distillation products.

3. Format of the experimental report

3.1 Purposes

3.2 Principle

3.3 The content of the experiment

3.4 Discussion

4. Considerations after the experiment

4.1 What is the role of radish in the process of mirabilite purification?

4.2 What is the principle of fermentation and germination methods?

4.3 Why is it necessary to control the appropriate bud length during germination?

4.4 What are the similarities and differences between the roasting method and stir-frying with solid adjuvant?

(Edited by Xiaolin Yang, Zhiguo Ma and Xiaoya Sun)

实验二十二 巴豆及其炮制品中巴豆油的含量测定

实验目的 •••

1. 掌握巴豆油的含量测定方法。
2. 了解巴豆霜中巴豆油含量与巴豆霜质量的关系。

实验原理 •••

巴豆（Crotonis Fructus）为大戟科植物巴豆 *Croton tiglium* L.的干燥成熟果实。外用蚀疮。用于恶疮疥癣、疣痣。巴豆有大毒，泻下猛烈，去油制霜后可降低毒性，缓和泻下作用，可用于峻下积滞，逐水消肿，豁痰利咽等。

巴豆油是巴豆泻下的有效成分，属于油脂类，不溶于水，易溶于有机溶剂，如苯、石油醚、乙醚、三氯甲烷等。选择溶剂时往往选择易溶出目的物且只溶出极少杂质而又易于除掉的溶剂，较为理想的溶剂有乙醚、石油醚。本实验对巴豆及巴豆霜进行巴豆油含量测定和比较。

实验器材 •••

1. **仪器** 索氏提取器，称量瓶，水浴锅，蒸发皿，干燥器等。
2. **药材及试剂** 巴豆（药材），无水乙醚，无水硫酸钠。

实验内容 •••

巴豆油的含量测定 取两只滤纸筒，分别装入适量的脱脂棉（用玻璃丝更佳），然后用表面皿精确称取巴豆霜及生巴豆泥各5g，小心放入滤纸筒内，注意切勿损失并用少量脱脂棉将附在表面皿上的药物搽净放入滤纸筒内，上盖适量的脱脂棉，然后将滤纸筒放入索氏提取器的提取管中，加入100mL乙醚，在水浴上加热至脂肪油提尽为止（若每小时回流7~8次，提取完全6~8小时），放冷后小心将滤纸筒取出（注意勿弄脏提取筒），利用原装置加热回收乙醚，然后将提取液倾入预先洗净干燥并已精确称量的蒸发皿中，并用少量无水乙醚洗涤小烧瓶，一并加入蒸发皿中，在水浴上徐徐蒸发，待乙醚去尽后，再放入干燥箱中，于100~105℃干燥1小时，移入干燥器中冷却半小时，精确称重，并计算生巴豆及巴豆霜中巴豆油的百分含量：

$$巴豆油的百分含量 = \frac{巴豆油重（mg）}{样品重（g）\times 1000} \times 100\%$$

实验指导 •••

1. 预习

（1）为什么要测巴豆霜中巴豆油的含量？

（2）怎样进行巴豆油的含量测定？

（3）测定巴豆油时为什么要选用乙醚为溶剂？

（4）炮制巴豆时，应该注意哪些安全防护措施？

2. 基本操作和操作注意点

（1）基本操作 正确进行巴豆油的含量测定。

（2）操作注意点 ①巴豆有大毒，操作时应戴口罩，操作后应用冷水洗手及用具，以防中毒。

②加入乙醚的量约占烧瓶容量的2/3，不宜过多或过少。③水浴中水温不宜过高（一般40~50℃为宜）。以免乙醚沸腾过剧，导致冷凝不完全而大量损失。④水浴不能用直火加热，以免引起乙醚燃烧，甚至爆炸，若水温太低可加沸水或更换热水。⑤样品不能直接放入提取管中，应盛于滤纸筒内，而且滤纸筒的底部要严密，上部也应用脱脂棉盖紧，以免样品进入烧瓶内，影响提取。⑥未提取时，冷凝管顶端可用软木塞塞紧，以免乙醚挥发掉，但提取时必须去掉。

3. 实验报告格式

（1）实验目的

（2）实验原理

（3）实验内容

（4）数据及计算结果

巴豆油含量测定

表22-1　巴豆油的含量

样品	样品重量（g）	油重（g）	百分含量（%）
生品			
炮制品			

（5）讨论

4. 实验后思考

（1）巴豆为什么要制霜后使用？《中国药典》规定巴豆霜中巴豆油含量范围是多少？

（2）巴豆中的毒性成分有哪几种？它们各自的特点是什么？怎样才能除掉或破坏这些成分？

（马志国　陆奕霜）

Experiment 22　The Assay of Croton Oil in the Crude and the Processed Crotonis Fructus

◆ Experimental purpose

1. To master the determination method for croton oil in Crotonis Fructus.

2. To learn about the relationship between the content of croton oil and the quality of Crotonis Semen Pulveratum(Badoushuang).

◆ Experimental principle

Crotonis Fructus is the dried ripe fruit of *Croton tiglium* L. (Fam. Euphorbiaceae). It could be used for phagedenic ulcer by external use, its indication is malignant ulcer, scabies and wart. It is highly poisonous, and has the drastic action of catharticizing. Both its toxicity and the drastically cathartic action are alleviated after removing the oil to take the kernel. The processed drug is used for dyspeptic disease, detumescence, eliminating phlegm for relieving sore-throat.

Croton oil is the effective ingredient in Crotonis Fructus. And it belongs to fats and oils, which are insoluble in water, but easy soluble in organic solvents, such as benzol, petroleum benzine, diethyl ether, chloroform and so on. Petroleum benzine and diethyl ether are the ideal solvent which could dissolve croton oil specifically and extra low impurity. This experiment uses diethyl ether as the solvent to extract the croton oil for the determination. This experiment first involves preparing Crotonis Semen Pulveratum, and then measuring and comparing the content of croton oil in Crotonis Fructus and Crotonis Semen Pulveratum.

◆ Experimental apparatus

1. Instruments

Soxhlet's apparatus, weighing flask, water both kettle, desiccators, evaporation dish.

2. Medicinal materials and chemicals

Crotonis Fructus(drug), anhydrous diethyl ether(C.P), Anhydrous Sodium Fulfate(C.P).

◆ Experimental content

Assay of croton oil of Crotonis Fructus

Put proper amount of absorbent cotton on the bottom of two filter paper tanks respectively. Weigh accurately 5g of crude Crotonis Fructus paste and Crotonis Semen Pulveratum to two filter paper tanks, respectively. Rubbed with a small amount of the absorbent cotton to avoid the loss. Add proper amount of absorbent cotton on the top of the tanks. Heat them in Soxhlet's apparatus with 100mL of the ether for 6-8 hours to exhaust croton oil. Allow it to stand cool, transfer the extract to the weighed evaporating dish, remove the ether at a low temperature on a water bath. Dry the residue at 100-105℃ for 1 hour, cool, and weigh it accurately. And calculate the content of croton oil in the drug.

$$\text{Content (\%)of croton oil} = \frac{W_{oil}}{W_{sample} \times 1000} \times 100\%$$

◆ Experimental instruction

1. Preview

1.1 Why determinate the content of croton oil in Crotonis Semen Pulveratum?

1.2 How to determinate the content of croton oil in the Crotonis Fructus?

1.3 Why is the ether used as the solvent when assaying the content of croton oil?

1.4 What protective actions should be taken when processing the Crotonis Fructus?

2. Primary operations and notes of operations

2.1 Primary operations

Master the determining method of croton oil.

2.2 Notes of operations

2.2.1 Wear mask when processing, because of the big toxicity of the drug. Make sure to wash your hands and instruments with cold water in case of poisoning.

2.2.2 The amount of the ether should not beyond 2/3 of the volume of the flask, neither too less.

2.2.3 The temperature of the water bath should not be too high (generally 40-50℃), otherwise the ether will boil drastically, and loss too much.

2.2.4 The ether cannot be heated directly on fire, otherwise it will cause the ether to burn and even explode fire even explosion. If the water temperature is too low, add boil water or change hot water.

2.2.5 The sample should be packed with filter paper rather than being put into the Soxhlet's extractor directly, or the sample powder will be put into the extractor to affect the extraction.

2.2.6 The topper of extractor could prevent the escaping of ether before extracting. But the stopper must be removed when extraction begins.

3. Format of experimental report

3.1 Purpose

3.2 Principle

3.3 The content of the experiment

3.4 Experimental data and calculating results

Assay of croton oil

Table 22-1　Assay of croton oil

Sample	Sample weight (g)	Oil weight (g)	Content (%)
Crude drug			
Processed drug			

3.5 Discussion

4. Considerations after the experiment

4.1 Why should the Crotonis Fructus be processed to the frost-like powder? What is the oil content range according to *The Pharmacopoeia of China*?

4.2 How many kinds of toxic components are there in the Crotonis Fructus? How to eliminate them?

（Edited by Zhiguo Ma and Yishuang Lu）

第九章 设计性实验

实验二十三 何首乌炮制研究设计性实验

设计性实验有别于传统的验证性实验。综合性与设计性是该类实验的主要特点。综合性体现在所涉及的实验内容不局限于中药炮制学，可以涵盖中药学专业各个专业领域，呈现实验内容复合性、实验手段与方法多样性的特点。设计性体现在实验是由教师指定实验项目的范围、实验目的和实验要求，但实验方案、实验条件、拟采用的技术与方法由学生自行设计，自主完成实验内容并对结果进行综合分析处理。设计性实验整个教学过程不仅要求学生综合多学科知识和多种实验原理、方法、手段来设计实验方案，还要求学生运用已有的专业知识去发现、分析和解决问题，其目的在于培养学生掌握科研设计实验的方法和步骤，激发学生学习的主动性、创造性，提高学生自主学习能力、认知能力，开拓学生的创新意识。

中药炮制设计性实验选题内容广泛，可以从不同炮制方法的比较研究、炮制工艺的优选研究、饮片质量的评价方法研究、饮片质量标准的研究、炮制前后化学成分的比较研究、传统炮制经验的科学内涵研究、炮制前后药效与毒性的对比研究等进行选题。但应遵循中医药理论，综合运用中药炮制、化学、药理学、数理统计等多学科知识，进行实验设计，充分体现其科学性、创新性，还应考虑所在实验室所具备的实验条件和实验成本，确保实验的可操作性和可行性。

实验目的 •••

1. 掌握中药炮制设计性实验的目的、要求与思路；文献查阅的方法、文献综述和科研论文的写作方法。
2. 通过实验掌握何首乌的炮制方法、原理和意义。
3. 提高对中药知识的综合应用能力，分析和解决问题的能力。
4. 通过分工开展各项实验设计和研究工作，培养学生的团队合作精神及协作意识。

选题思路 •••

结合实验室现有的实验条件和学时安排，可从以下4个方向进行选题：

1. 何首乌的炮制方法 何首乌饮片的炮制方法中未见水处理软化的工艺参数，切制规格包括厚片和块。文献报道制何首乌的炮制方法有清蒸和黑豆汁蒸两种蒸制方法、常压蒸和加压蒸两种加热方式，也有九蒸九晒的传统工艺，各方法制备的制何首乌饮片功效与质量有无差别？何首乌蒸制时要求使用非铁质容器，有无实验证实其原因？

2. 何首乌生品、制品的质量评价 饮片外观性状与其内在质量之间是否存在关联性？如何用现代技术客观表征饮片颜色、气味等传统主观评价指标？二苯乙烯苷类、蒽醌类成分含量高低能否表明其有效性？有无更科学的何首乌饮片质量评价方法？

3. 何首乌生品、制品的药效评价 文献资料表明，何首乌的炮制原理不仅仅体现在增效上，还体现在降低不良反应，主要指生品的急性肝损伤和对胃肠道的刺激引起腹泻等不良反应。已采用的实验方法有哪些？如何设计才能体现在中医药理论指导下开展实验研究？

4. 何首乌生品、制品的药性评价 中药炮生为熟引起的药性改变与其内在物质基础的变化有关。

内在物质基础的变化包括量变和质变，单纯一种成分的变化并不能全面解释整个单味中药饮片功效的改变。在查阅文献时需注意采用什么方法能够基本表明炮制前后的物质基础变化情况，如何选择药效指标研究生品、制品的功效改变，阐明其炮制程度与药性改变的关系，寻找其质量标志物，进一步探讨其炮制原理。

实验要求

1. 通过对何首乌炮制方法及工艺研究的设计，掌握中药炮制方法及工艺优选的基本方法与思路。
2. 通过对何首乌饮片质量研究的设计，掌握传统与现代中药饮片质量评价方法与思路。
3. 通过对何首乌生品和制品毒性、功效比较研究的设计，掌握何首乌饮片的主要药效、毒理学评价方法与思路。

实验内容

1. 文献查阅与综述的撰写　通过查阅《中国药典》、各地《炮制规范》和何首乌研究文献资料，撰写何首乌饮片炮制研究进展综述，分析何首乌的炮制工艺、饮片质量评价、药理与临床、炮制机制研究的现状及发展趋势，找出存在的问题，明确研究目标，为实验方案设计奠定基础。

2. 制定实验方案　根据选课人数将学生分为若干组，每组3~5人。各组在综合整理何首乌炮制相关文献的基础上，进行选题，确定研究方向。根据设计性实验的要求，应用所学的中药学专业知识围绕研究目标拟定实验方案，论证方案的可行性，分析实验中可能出现的问题，形成设计方案初稿。设计报告应包括：课题名称、选题依据、研究目的、实验原理、仪器与试药、实验内容、预期结果、可能遇到的问题、参考文献等。各小组汇报实验方案，教师组织学生听取汇报，并对设计方案从创新性、可行性等方面进行引导性评价，各小组根据教师的意见对设计方案进行修改，完成实验方案的制定。

3. 实验实施　各组整理实验用仪器、试药清单，实验室、仪器使用计划，按时提交给实验室管理员，用于实验准备。学生按照实验计划开展实验，并做好实验记录。实验过程中遇到的问题及时与教师、实验室管理员沟通解决，及时调整优化实验方案。

4. 实验总结与报告提交　学生根据原始记录，分析、归纳、整理实验数据，讨论实验结果、实验中遇到的主要问题及解决办法，并撰写实验报告。实验报告撰写要求：①参照科研论文体例撰写；②对照设计报告说明完成情况，如未完成，应说明原因；③实验结论应符合逻辑，结果可信，根据结果客观分析、讨论，保持科学严谨的态度，总结经验教训和学习心得。

5. 总结汇报　同组同学对整个实验过程进行自我评价；各组分别汇报，不同组同学之间讨论交流；指导教师从实验报告、原始记录、总结汇报中找出普遍存在的问题集中点评，并对各组从设计报告、实验过程与结果、实验报告、总结汇报等方面综合给予评价。

注意事项

1. 每组同学可选定本实验项下的单一研究方向进行实验设计。所设计的实验方案需合理可行，注意细节性及可操作性，需附参考文献作为支撑材料。
2. 实验方案中的工艺、质量、药效等评价指标，应充分体现与何首乌生、制品的功能主治相一致的原则。

思考题

1. 简述中药炮制研究的方法与思路。
2. 简述中药炮制研究的方向与进展。

（马志国　陆奕霜）

Experiment 23   Design Experiment on the Processing of Polygoni Multiflori Radix

The design experiments are different from the traditional Chinese medicine processing experiment. The main characteristics of this type of experiment are comprehensiveness and designability. The comprehensiveness is reflected in that the experiment content is not limited to the traditional Chinese medicine processing, but has been extended to various professional fields. Therefore, it has the characteristics of complex experimental content and diverse experimental methods. The designability is shown in that the teacher specifies the scope, purposes and requirements of the experiment, while the students design the experimental scheme, determine the experimental conditions, technologies and methods, complete the experimental content and comprehensively analyze and process the results independently. The entire teaching process of design experiments not only requires students to integrate multidisciplinary knowledge and various experimental principles, methods, and means to design experimental plans, but also requires them to use their existing professional knowledge to discover, analyze, and solve problems. The purpose is to cultivate students' mastery of the methods and steps of scientific research design experiments, stimulate students' initiative and creativity in learning, improve their self-learning and cognitive abilities, and expand students' innovative awareness.

The topic selection of design experiments for traditional Chinese medicine processing is extensive, including comparative research on different processing methods, optimization of processing techniques, evaluation methods for the quality of decoction pieces, quality standards for decoction pieces, comparison of chemical components before and after processing, scientific connotation research on traditional processing experience, and comparative research on efficacy and toxicity before and after processing. However, it is necessary to follow the theory of traditional Chinese medicine, comprehensively use multidisciplinary knowledge such as Chinese medicine processing, chemistry, pharmacology, mathematical statistics, and carry out experimental design to fully reflect its scientificity and innovation. It is also necessary to consider the experimental conditions and costs of the laboratory to ensure the operability and feasibility of the experiment.

◆ Experimental purposes

1. To master the purposes, requirements, and ideas of design experiments for traditional Chinese medicine (TCM) processing. To master the methods for searching and collecting related references in literature, writing reviews and scientific papers.

2. To master the processing methods, principles and significance of Polygoni Multiflori Radix through performing the experiment.

3. To improve students' comprehensive abilities in TCM and the abilities to analyze and solve problems.

4. To train and promote team spirit and cooperative consciousness through designing related experiments.

◆ Topic selection ideas

Based on the existing experimental conditions and schedules in the laboratory, topics can be selected from the following four directions:

1. The methods for processing Polygoni Multiflori Radix

There is no process parameter for water treatment softening in the processing method of Polygoni Multiflori Radix, and the cutting specifications include thick slices and blocks. It has been reported in the literature that the processing methods of Polygoni Multiflori Radix include two steaming methods like steaming and steaming with black bean juice, and two heating methods, such as atmospheric steam and pressurized steam. There are also some traditional processes, like nine kinds of steaming and drying respectively. Are there any differences in the efficacy and quality of Polygoni Multiflori Radix prepared by various methods? Does any experiment confirm the reason why nonferrous containers are required for the steaming of Polygoni Multiflori Radix?

2. Quality evaluation of raw and processed Polygoni Multiflori Radix

Is there a correlation between the appearance and internal quality of decoction pieces? How to use modern technology to objectively characterize traditional subjective evaluation indicators such as the color and odor of decoction pieces? Can the content of stilbene glycosides and anthraquinone components indicate their effectiveness? Is there a more scientific method for evaluating the quality of Polygoni Multiflori Radix?

3. Pharmacodynamic evaluation of raw and processed Polygoni Multiflori Radix

Literature shows that the processing principle of Polygoni Multiflori Radix is not only reflected in enhancing efficacy, but also in reducing toxicity and side effects, mainly referring to the acute liver injury caused by raw materials and diarrhea caused by gastrointestinal stimulation. What the experimental methods have been used? How to design experimental research that can be reflected under the guidance of traditional Chinese medicine theory?

4. Pharmacological evaluation of raw and processed Polygoni Multiflori Radix

The changes in medicinal properties caused by the maturation of traditional Chinese medicine are related to the changes in its internal material basis. The changes in the internal material basis include both quantitative and qualitative changes, and a single component change alone cannot fully explain the changes in the efficacy of a single traditional Chinese medicine decoction. When consulting literature, it is necessary to pay attention to the methods used to study the changes in the material base before and after processing, which can basically indicate the changes in the material base before and after processing. How to select efficacy indicators to study the efficacy changes of raw and processed products, clarify the relationship between the degree of processing and the changes in drug properties, search for quality markers, and further explore their processing principles.

◆ Experimental requirements

1. Through the design of processing methods and processes for Polygoni Multiflori Radix, grasp the basic methods and ideas for optimizing traditional Chinese medicine processing methods and processes.

2. By designing research on the quality of prepared Polygoni Multiflori Radix, master the methods and ideas for evaluating the quality of traditional and modern Chinese medicine decoction pieces.

3. Through the design of comparative studies on the toxicity and efficacy of raw and processed Polygoni Multiflori Radix, grasp the main pharmacological and toxicological evaluation methods and ideas of Polygoni Multiflori Radix.

◆ Experimental contents

1. Literature review and writing of reviews

By consulting the Chinese Pharmacopoeia, local processing standards and research literature on Polygoni Multiflori Radix, a review of the research progress in the processing of Polygoni Multiflori Radix decoction pieces is written. The current status and development trend of the processing technology, quality evaluation of decoction pieces, pharmacology and clinical studies, and processing mechanism research of Polygoni Multiflori Radix are analyzed to identify existing problems, clarify research objectives, and lay the foundation for experimental scheme design.

2. Develop experimental plan

Divide students into several groups based on the number of course participants, with 3-5 students in each group. On the basis of comprehensively organizing relevant literature on the processing of Polygoni Multiflori Radix, each group selected topics and determined research directions. According to the requirements of design experiments, apply the professional knowledge of traditional Chinese medicine learned to develop experimental plans around the research objectives, demonstrate the feasibility of the plans, analyze possible problems in the experiments, and form the first draft of the design plan. The design report should include: project name, topic selection basis, research purpose, experimental principle, instruments and drugs, experimental content, expected results, potential problems encountered, references, etc. Each group reports on the experimental plan, the teacher organizes students to listen to the report, and makes a guided evaluation of the design plan in terms of innovation, feasibility, and other aspects. Each group modifies the plan based on the teacher's opinions and completes the formulation of the experimental plan.

3. Experimental implementation

Each group shall compile a list of experimental instruments and drugs, as well as a plan for the use of laboratory and instruments, and submit it to the laboratory administrator on time for experimental preparation. Students carry out experiments according to the experimental plan and keep experimental records. Communicate with teachers and laboratory administrators in a timely manner to solve any problems encountered during the experiment, and adjust and optimize the experimental plan in time.

4. Experimental summary and report submission

Students analyze, summarize, and organize experimental data based on original records, discuss experimental results, main problems encountered in the experiment, and solutions, and write experimental reports. Requirements for writing experimental reports: Firstly, write according to the style of scientific research papers; Secondly, compare the completion status with the design report, and if not completed, explain the reason; Thirdly, the experimental conclusion should be logical, the results credible, objectively analyzed and discussed based on the results, maintain a scientific and rigorous attitude, summarize lessons learning experiences.

5. Summary and report

Self-evaluation of the entire experimental process by classmates in the same group; Each group reports separately, and students from different groups discuss and exchange ideas; Guide teachers to identify common problems from experimental reports, original records, and summary reports, and provide comprehensive comments for each group from aspects such as design reports, experimental processes and results, experimental reports, and summary reports.

◆ Notes

1. Each group of students can choose a single research direction under this experimental project for experimental design. The designed experimental plan should be reasonable and feasible, pay attention to details and operability, and attach reference materials as supporting materials.

2. The evaluation indicators such as process, quality, and efficacy in the experimental plan should fully reflect the principle of consistency with the functional indications of Polygoni Multiflori Radix raw and processed products.

◆ Question

1. Briefly describe the methods and ideas of traditional Chinese medicine processing research.

2. Briefly describe the direction and progress of research on traditional Chinese medicine processing.

（Edited by Zhiguo Ma and Yishuang Lu）